Awkwardly Strong

&

By Paula Jean Ferri

TABLE OF CONTENTS

Introduction

Chapter 1   My Story

Chapter 2   Background

Chapter 3   Current Struggles for Individuals with TS

Chapter 4   How to Be the Author of Your Life Story

Chapter 5   Conclusion

Appendix A   Supporting Individuals with TS

Appendix B   Resources

References

Acknowledgements

About the Author

INTRODUCTION

I sat there tapping my foot on the perfectly polished marble floor. I could feel the quiet reverence of the place, even if I wasn't completely a part of the silence. I've just never been the type of person who can sit still. And I certainly can't sit still and be quiet.

Sometimes I just let out a scream, and there's really no good reason for it. It just kind of happens. And it's the most entertaining thing, and one of my favorite things, about myself.

One of those screams came out that day as I was in the Salt Lake City Temple (a quiet place of learning and reflection). I was in the cafeteria when I saw my stake president walk into the room. (For those of you who aren't familiar with the term "stake president," he's basically the equivalent of, say, a priest, minister, rabbi, etc. in other faiths. My point is that he's someone I knew and respected and someone I was happy to see.) Without thinking, I shouted out with joy and caused a little bit of commotion with my enthusiastic greeting. After I settled down a bit, I said hello to him.

That's when another person, a respected leader in the church, in fact, leaned around the corner and said, "Please remember where you are."

Now, I knew he didn't know who I was or know about my background, so I wasn't offended. I simply informed him that I had Tourette Syndrome, and he instantly apologized.

Awkwardly Strong

This is why I can never sit still. My tics keep me moving more often than I would like and cause me to scream and make random noises without my control or permission. My Tourette Syndrome (TS) certainly knows how to keep me on my toes, since I never know exactly what will come out of my own mouth.

Normally my TS is pretty respectful in the temple—we seem to have an understanding, my Tourette's and me, about how to behave. I know I can't control it, but for the most part, I can live with it. My TS is just a part of my life—a part of me like the color of my eyes or the size of my feet. So we get along ok. It works out.

That day in the temple, however, my Tourette's wasn't so in line. But throughout the years, I've learned how to live with, and embrace, my TS, and I've realized that it's ok that I sometimes scream and that I can't sit still and that I'm simply a unique individual with my own quirks, just like everyone else.

Looking back now, I actually value this experience in the Salt Lake temple. What I loved about this interaction (other than the fact that my TS helped me rub elbows with such an important person!) was that this gentleman was instantly worried about having offending me and he made sure that I still felt loved after the incident. He told me, "That's great. Well, not great that you have Tourette Syndrome, but great that you let me know!" I simply laughed and said, "Really? I think it's quite great!"

He has a medical background, so he let me know that he knows what Tourette's is and that he understood, so we got to skip the medical discussion that I sometimes have to have with people when I'm explaining why I make noises. He was so sweet about the whole thing, even putting his arms around me in a great hug.

I guess having Tourette Syndrome has its advantages.

※

I count myself lucky that I've had such positive experiences like this with my TS. But not everyone is that fortunate these days. On the contrary, people are becoming more and more detached from one another in these kinds of situations, and in relationships in general. Fewer relationships stand the test of time, and it grows ever harder to even know how to make friends. We see this in memes on the Internet and in our own awkward complaints of making friends after thirty.

To make matters worse, there is a growing issue of neurological idiosyncrasies, like TS, constantly throwing a wrench into the works of being social. This group of people with brains wired differently will struggle more than the average person in social areas. We have quirks that make us seem weird, and sometimes those quirks make us stand out. Many people can see right away that we are unusual, but few really understand why. And not feeling understood is a quick way to feel disconnected.

The good news is that we don't have to feel that way. We can fully enjoy the people around us and all of life's opportunities that come with building relationships. In this book, I'll teach you how to significantly multiply the relationships in your life, both in quality and quantity, or whichever best suits you. In fact, you may become good at social relationships because of your differences, rather than despite them. People with idiosyncrasies have an advantage, quite frankly, and that power can be both thrilling and exciting, and sometimes even terrifying.

In this book, I'll outline information about these neurological quirks that I've mentioned and discuss how to overcome the difficulties of being social in today's world, beyond just the differences of the mind. This book will open your eyes to see social interaction as more than a fearsome experience, and I'll help you improve your communication and relationships and, hopefully, create new ones!

When you're finished reading this book, I want you to have the confidence to create the relationships and social life you desire. My goal is that you won't feel held back by your differences and the awkwardness you typically feel in social situations but, instead, feel empowered to write the story of your life as you want it to be written.

There's one thing to especially keep in mind as you read this book: one of the most important tools we have for cultivating relationships is time. We are only given so much time on this earth, so I encourage you to begin now to create and nourish friendships. Rather than regretting in the future the lost time with those you loved, and with people in general, take the time today. Why wait to start?

My Story

I started making noises when I was 17. The very first noise came while I was at work one day at our local library (yes, of all places, a library). I happened to be in the back room, and I was alone when it happened. I made a funny little noise—one that sounded like a squeaky toy (hence the reason I started calling them "squeaks"). I thought it was interesting, kind of like a hiccup, but it didn't hurt and I only did one. So I didn't take much notice. However, I did one again the following day, also at work. This time I was around some of the ladies who worked at the library. They thought it was a cute little noise, and life went on.

Once the noises started, I had quite a few interesting experiences with them, but as I don't remember any of them being negative, I just lived on as any person without them would. In my mind I was normal—the noises were simply something that happened every once in a while, just like a hiccup or a sneeze. It was always the same little sound, and it just wasn't a big deal.

And then the noises started happening every day. The library ladies still thought it was adorable, so we usually had a nice little chuckle when they happened. I don't know how long it went on like that, but soon I started doing it more than once a day. It was my coworker Connie who started to realize I was doing them more often and started counting how many noises I made during my shift. Once she started counting, the noises became more frequent. We still had chuckles over it, and I wasn't too concerned, mostly because, as I mentioned before, it didn't hurt to make the noises. I don't feel anything when I make them.

The noises continued, and high school continued on pretty much like normal. During high school I discovered music and choir, and I fell in love with them. I wanted to become a choir director. So when I graduated from high school, I went on to Snow College as a music major, and my life was right on track.

But while I was at Snow, things started to change. I started doing two noises in a row anytime I made them, and I made the noises multiple times a day. My parents were, understandably, concerned, maybe more than I was, and had me visit the family doctor. I didn't squeak at all during the visit, but after explaining the noises to the doctor, the doctor said that it was something I should see a specialist about.

Overall, I ended up seeing three different doctors. All of them, in different ways, told me they didn't know what was going on…

※

During my second year at Snow, I started doing sets of three squeaks. So, as you can imagine, the noises started getting more attention, and I started getting reactions from people. Now as a voice emphasis, I started studying the different problems that can harm a vocalist, and at about that same time, I was in a school production called MAME. I was only in the chorus, but I started to have a constant sore throat from all the strain. I decided to see a doctor about my constant sore throat, and my voice teacher recommended a doctor for me.

During my visit, I brought up the squeaks. The doctor tested my blood (I'm terrified of needles, so I wasn't too happy with that idea), but nothing came back and the doctor was stumped.

Time passed, the squeaks continued, and I graduated from Snow with my associate's degree. After that I moved home and went to an ear, nose, and throat doctor. Like the other doctors I'd seen over the years, he said he had never heard of anything like my squeaks and didn't know how to help.

At one point, since no one was quite able to diagnose what I was going through, one of the doctors gave me some things to do for my sore throat and said that something had to be spasming to create a noise like that, so he also gave me some muscle relaxant. The next day, I took the muscle relaxant. About an hour after taking it, I squeaked. So much for that theory…

One night, I did four squeaks in a row, and this was the first time I really started to get concerned. If this was going to be a pattern, it might become a problem. I only did four in a row once, though. After that night, the cute little squeaks started to…evolve. Some got longer, and they started to fluctuate in pitch. There were small differences at first, but as more time passed, the more the noises changed. Most of the time I still had my cute little hiccup-like squeak, but every once in a while, the noises were different.

At some point, despite my changing squeaks, I realized that I couldn't live my life worrying about them, especially when numerous doctors didn't have answers about what I was going through. So I stopped worrying about the noises, and I turned in my mission papers. Mission papers are like an application saying I want to complete a period of service for the Church of Jesus

Christ of Latter-day Saints, and these papers help determine the best mission for each person based on any health concerns, etc. So I knew I would be assigned to a mission that would work for me personally. And it was; I went on my mission and had several great experiences.

About halfway through my mission, the mission doctor, Dr. Dahl, came to visit and heard one of my squeaks. One of the originals. I apologized and told him I didn't know what it was; it was just something I do. He said, "I bet it is Tourette's. You would have to do some neurological tests, but I'm pretty sure that is what it would be." Other people had suggested that before, so I had heard the term, but I didn't really know what it was, just that it really didn't have a cure.

My reaction to Dr. Dahl? Why would I pay an extravagant amount of money for someone to tell me there is no cure for what I was going through? I was comfortable with my squeaks, so I just let the idea roll off my back.

&

Fast forward three years later: I was studying to get my bachelor's degree in social work. I still made noises, but other than that, I was just your average college student. One day, however, I was pulled aside by my professors and was told that with these noises, they could not place me in an internship. As an internship was required for graduation, they were basically telling me that I would need to find a new major…

And that was the last straw.

Having overloaded myself with work and extracurricular activities, I simply gave up trying to keep up with class work. I had to find a new major anyway, right? What was the point of trying so hard at school when I couldn't study what I felt I was called to, especially when I was rejected from the program because of something I had no control over? After that tough news, it was hard for me to bounce back. My grades started slipping, and I failed my classes that semester.

So I had to pick a new major. It wasn't an easy decision, but I knew I wanted to earn my bachelor's, and I knew there had to be something else out there that I could enjoy studying. Eventually I decided on international cultural studies with an emphasis in communications. Before I could start though, I needed to see one of the school counselors to make sure I was okay and in a position where I would not fail all of my classes again.

After explaining the noises that I make and my experience in the social work department, I was officially diagnosed with TS by Dr. Orr, the school psychologist at the BYUH campus. I was 24 years old. I didn't have much of a reaction to finally receiving a diagnosis, despite seven years of noises. I was grateful to finally have a name for it—mostly for those few people who would try to "fix" me when they heard my noises. They would ask question after question, "Have you tried this? Have you tried that? Is it this?" After so many questions, I had been telling them it was Tourette Syndrome just to stop it, even years before the official diagnosis. It was no surprise to me.

&♥

Throughout the rest of my college career, I learned a lot about TS, and I learned even more about myself. I loved the major I had chosen, and the things I learned in college have been of infinite value to me and my understanding of myself and the people around me. I felt extremely validated for all the weird thoughts and habits I had even as a child.

These are the epiphanies I wish to share with you. I am so often heartbroken by people who are scared or ignorant of neurological quirks like TS. You'll notice I will never, EVER call these quirks "disabilities." People with these quirks are in no way, shape, or form disabled. We are different and have our strengths and our weaknesses, just like anyone else.

I have found that having TS has opened more doors for me than closing them. I have more relationships because of my TS, and those relationships are more open, despite being ridiculously awkward. Throughout the years, and especially since I was diagnosed with TS, I have learned many tricks and secrets as I've studied people and how they communicate. I don't want these observations to be secrets to you. I don't want you to have to pay thousands of dollars, or take years of study (as I did), to learn how to improve your communication. Instead, take it from someone who's walked a mile in your shoes—someone in the same position as you.

You may have quirks—everyone does—and these are the things that make you an individual. Your quirks don't have to hold you back or limit your life in any way. On the contrary, these quirks can work to your advantage.

You can improve your communication skills. You can improve your relationships. You can take control and be the author of your own life story.

Take these tips and tricks that I've learned and use them to write the story of your life.

I'll show you how.

Background

I am often amazed by how many people have never heard of TS, so I want to take this chapter to discuss what I've learned about Tourette Syndrome and how it works, as well as touch a little on the spectrum that it's a part of. After all, the first step in addressing any issue is to fully understand what you're facing. Without that, how do you figure out how to get around it? Better yet, how do you figure out how to get through it?

So, let's talk about TS.

Definition

For people with TS or other neurological quirks, our brains work a little differently from people without those quirks. Although there are many theories about Tourette Syndrome, my favorite theory (and the theory that, based on research, is most like my brain) is that it's on the same spectrum of neurological oddities as Autism, Asperger's, Attention Deficit Disorder (ADD), and Obsessive-Compulsive Disorder (OCD). People with these disorders struggle in their own little way with social interaction. There are several types of TS, and some forms of TS claim no relation at all to this spectrum, even though ADD and OCD are often diagnosed along with TS. But nothing is proven. TS is often explained in literature as a "brain disorder characterized by different types of tics" (Peters 2009, 14). TS usually contains at least one physical and one vocal tic, and tics vary by individual.

For example, one person may have Coprolalia, the rare but well-known stereotype of TS, where the individual swears or yells other obscenities, while another individual may bark or scream as a vocal tic. Others may have a form known as Echolalia, where they echo noises, words, or phrases they hear around them. Individuals with TS can also have multiple tics, making the same person do both a shoulder twitch and walk in circles as a motor tic.

When I tell people I have Tourette Syndrome, 9 times out of 10, they respond with, "So, you swear and stuff?" (Coprolalia). Out of all the people who have TS (and really, how many do you know?), only 1 in 10 has Coprolalia. Echolalia, the kind of TS that I have, is just as uncommon. These are the only forms of TS that have a classification, as most tics vary so much in individuals.

My tics tend to lean toward echoing noises I hear often, but the noises are always different and are rarely a direct echo. For instance, I mimic the noises of the time clock at work, various animals, and ghosts, and I even "sing" along to songs, sometimes songs that I didn't even know that I knew.

I never know what is going to come out of my mouth. It's as much of a surprise to me as it is to everyone else around me, and I'm sure many people who have TS feel the same way.

This brings us to a very important character in this book: Jess (a.k.a., my TS). With my TS having such a mind of its own, I decided to just embrace the situation and give my TS a name: Jess. As you read on, you'll notice that Jess has quite a few stories of her own, and she'll tell you all about them.

Anyway, tics are a large part of TS, and once I learned more about TS and how my squeaks, or "tics" as I now know they're called, were an actual "thing," I started to realize just how often these tics actually happen in my life. Not only that, but how long I have been having tics, even before I realized I had TS. For instance, if you have ever watched a movie with me, you know that I repeat lines in the movie. This may not be a common tic, but for those with Echolalia, there might be something similar. Someone commented on it once, so I tried to make a conscious effort to stop. I thought it would be a simple habit to break. Then I started to realize how often I repeat things, not just from movies.

Even being aware of it, I still do it. Now that I'm aware of it though, I just make an effort to be more quiet when I do it. The weird part is that it sounds like me doing it, not even like Jess. She does it in her own way, but during movies it is not Jess's voice, so this tic was harder to catch.

Echolalia is something Jess does as well, though. Jess evolves as time passes, which is pretty typical of TS; she learns more "phrases." She mimics the tune of "I know something you don't know" and can say "Thank you." Every time Jess "speaks," it's the word "meh" and very high pitched, but always to the right tone and rhythm of how we would say a phrase. She has started saying words as well, from "Weeeee!" to "Whoa!" and even the occasional, "Yeah!" She even manages to stay in context too.

History

TS is also known as "Gilles de la Tourette's Syndrome." It was named after the French physician who first mentioned the possibility of these symptoms (vocal and verbal tics) being connected to each other, yet distinct from other known conditions. The creation of a diagnosis separate from other conditions was done back in 1885, so while Tourette Syndrome is not a new condition, it is still relatively unknown. In fact, some reports state that several victims in the Salem Witch Trials (from 1692–1693) might have simply had TS. There are records dating back to the ancient Greeks of symptoms that sound an awful lot like what we now call Tourette Syndrome. (Brill 2012, 33)

Since 1885 when the condition was named, TS has had a long history of stereotyping and misunderstandings. Marquise de Dampierre was a French woman gossiped about for most of her life in the early 1800s and is among the first people known to have TS. Her case was recorded by Jean Marc Gaspard Itard, who was best known for his work with the deaf and the invention of the catheter. He was also the first person to describe the symptoms of TS. He published a description of her and her fear of her own outbursts (she had Coprolalia), and sixty years later, George Gilles de la Tourette classified her case as maladie des tics. As this was a new diagnosis, it was named after Gilles de la Tourette (Kushner 2000).

Itard and others, in the sixty years before Gilles de la Tourette, thought that the outbursts were caused by external factors, rather than a neurological disorder, and could be cured. Itard believed that the men who showed symptoms of what is now known as Tourette's had merely "suffered from some irreversible organic brain damage" (Kushner 2000, 15).

He assumed women showing the same symptoms, however, had somehow not been taught correctly how to fulfill their roles in society as wives and mothers. He even believed that he had cured one young woman after five weeks of treatment. This may be possible, but other sources describe how the symptoms of TS come and go in phases, so the young woman may have just been in a phase where her symptoms were milder. Even now, the fact that symptoms are irregularly spaced makes it hard to target a direct link to any emotional or psychological factors as a trigger; however, the spacing itself is part of the list doctors check to diagnose TS (Spitzer 1994).

Statistics in the United States

TS typically appears around ages four to five (Centers for Disease Control and Prevention [CDCP] 2011). Due to the difficulty of diagnosing TS, it is unknown how many children actually have it; however, approximately 3 out of every 1,000 individuals between the ages of 6 to 17 have TS. Also, about 75 percent of these individuals are male (CDCP 2011), but it is unknown why males are more affected than females.

Another interesting note about TS: while all ethnic groups and races can be affected by TS, Caucasian, peoples are twice as likely to be diagnosed as Hispanics or African-Americans. However, there are not yet any theories to support the idea that TS is connected in any way to race. Over 33 percent of individuals with TS are also diagnosed with OCD and 79 percent are diagnosed with "at least one additional mental health, behavioral or developmental condition" (CDCP 2011).

TS is a chronic disorder. Symptoms typically will decrease with age, possibly with an understanding of how TS works and what can trigger more severe outbursts. And with no known cure for TS, only suggestions to diminish tics are available. However, the reactions to treatments vary from individual to individual. In any case, often a psychologist is seen, whether as treatment, or just to deal with living in a culture where no one understands what is going on.

Diagnosis

Tourette's was once thought of as a psychological problem, and those diagnosed were sent to psychoanalysis and psychotherapy (Kushner 2000, 45). My friend Emma, for instance, was sent to a psychologist by her family doctor to see whether she had TS. He did diagnose her with TS, but he thought that she was being abused in some form and pressed her with questions about her relationship with her parents. That idea has since been abandoned in Emma's case (Personal interview with Emma Hardy 2012).

People with TS have also been thought to be possessed by the devil (a thought that is, unfortunately, still alive and circulating—see The Landover Baptist Church Forum comment titled "Camp twitch and shout, camp for demon infested kids!" posted by Eliot Mayfield in June 2009) as well as being thought of as just plain weird. There are no official tests that can be run to discover whether an individual has TS, but a diagnosis can be given by a certified doctor, including psychologists or psychiatrists, in addition to medical doctors. TS can be hard to recognize due to other disorders that tend to go hand in hand with it and that are typically more well-known, such as Autism, Asperger's, OCD, ADD, or ADHD. People with TS often report depression, anxiety, and sometimes anger issues.

Many people see several doctors before getting a diagnosis. Due to a lack of any specific examination for TS, many doctors do not even think of the possibility. As I mentioned in Chapter 1, I saw three different doctors who had no idea what was going on before I was diagnosed with TS. Once TS has been diagnosed, it is watched for due to a possibility of TS being a genetic disorder (Comings 1990, 41). If a parent has TS, a son is 58 percent more likely to also have TS, and the chance of a daughter also having TS is 30 percent.

Treatment

It is unclear what exactly causes TS, which makes finding a "cure" rather difficult. Treatments can range anywhere from diet and exercise to medication and even extend by some to exorcism. As you can see, the treatment depends on what one considers to be the cause.

Some books, for instance, suggest alternative healing processes and natural treatments for TS (e.g., see Natural Treatments for Tics & Tourette's: A Patient and Family Guide by Sheila Rogers). In these books, the focus is on finding what "triggers" the tics in the body. Theories range from diet and allergies to "the toxic impact of heavy metals" (Buzbuzian 2007, 5) and other environmental factors. I read about one case where a mother described how these natural remedies "cured" her son. Meanwhile, some doctors recommend medicine as a treatment for Tourette's. Drugs most often used are Haloperidol, Pimozide, Clonidine, or even stimulants. However, many question the effectiveness of these drugs and seek more natural healing treatments.

Living with TS

Within the mental spectrum of TS, one of the many commonalities is that of difficulty in social settings. Our brains function on a different level, making it difficult to understand social cues. TS plays with these social cues and totally throws things off, but living with TS can still end up in your favor.

In the next chapters, I'll explore some of the other common struggles of living with TS, and once you understand what you're facing, I'll share with you how you can work through these challenges, face your unique quirks head-on, and take control of your life.

Current Struggles for Individuals with TS

Challenges Associated with Diagnosis

Living with TS, in itself, presents its own challenges, but it can become easier once you know what you're dealing with. However, even diagnosing TS is sometimes difficult. As I mentioned in Chapter 1, I wasn't diagnosed till I was 24!

So, let's talk a little bit about the challenges associated with diagnosis.

First, it's important to understand that TS is no respecter of persons. It will affect people of all ages. Typically, it will start around the age of four to five, so when we think of TS, we generally think of children. This is likely because of how much it can affect a child's view of the world and the child's view of himself or herself. A child with TS who may yet be undiagnosed (which is most children) is often told to stop being disruptive or is labeled as a "bad kid."

This labeling can drastically affect children's behavior if they think they really are "bad." Sometimes children may even develop a guilt complex, which can be very similar to depression. They might think that even when they try to be good, they end up doing bad things.

If the outside world and those close to a child reinforce that message, and if the child tries to stop the "bad" actions but can't and continues to get reprimanded, the child may become angry at the world and be unable to develop trust in other future relationships. The child might even start to own that "bad" label and continue being disruptive, but eventually the child's actions become intentional rather than something the child can't control.

How often do we, even as adults, give in to labels (e.g., "I'm fat," "I'm stupid," or "I'm not good enough")? And we buy in to these labels when we're old enough to recognize that not everything that people tell us is true. So imagine how much more of an impact labeling has on a child. Children are impressionable; they absorb information left and right, and when someone tells them they're "bad," they may not question it the way an adult would.

From the first appearance of symptoms of TS and throughout the diagnosis, a child's identity (or the identity of whomever is showing symptoms, including adults) can shift and change. One day a child may feel like any other child, and then the next day, the child's parents may start to notice the child doing something that other children don't do. A growl in the throat…Excessive eye blinking…An unfamiliar twitching of the shoulder…The parents may ask the child to stop, and the child may stop the action for a while, but the behavior persists.

Now what? How does the family react? Without a diagnosis, the child is left confused as to what is expected of him or her, the parents are concerned about the child's behavior or are upset that the child isn't listening, and the family is left feeling disconnected.

This kind of situation does happen, but not all children have to live with undiagnosed TS, and an early diagnosis can make all the difference. In Tic Talk: Living with Tourette Syndrome: A 9-year-old Boy's True Story about Living with Tourette Syndrome (2009), the author, Dylan Peters, describes his experience with TS. After several doctor trips and a diagnosis at a young age, Dylan's struggles allowed him to become a published author at the age of nine.

Another author with TS, Brad Cohen, shares his story of an inspirational teacher who changed his life (Cohen and Wysocky 2008). Brad discusses how this teacher inspired him to become a teacher as well, despite the fact that he had to overcome incredible odds, and many people told him he could never, and should never, be a teacher. Brad's journey with TS also started out as a struggle, but eventually he learned to live with it. He says of his TS, "I have learned that Tourette's is not always a hindrance; the coping skills Tourette Syndrome forced me to learn have also given me confidence to make my dream of being an effective and compassionate teacher a reality… without it [my Tourette Syndrome] I just wouldn't be me. Has it been a struggle? Of course. Has it been rewarding? Absolutely" (Cohen and Wysocky 2008, xiv).

People have often told me how well I seem to handle having TS. I personally think this is due to the fact that I developed TS as a teenager rather than in my young formative years. As a teenager with TS, there is more understanding of what is going on in the body. We have an idea of what we can control and what we can't. Children may have no idea what is going on, but teenagers have more of a grasp of the situation. The problem is that teenagers with more extreme cases of TS may still be influenced by the thoughts of those around them. Although teenagers are less impressionable than children, teenagers also tend to experience a great deal of peer pressure and worry more about what other people think of them. A teenager's tics, and the way that others react to those tics, can still affect the teenager's view of himself or herself and of the world around him or her.

When I started having my tics, I already knew I was a "good" kid, and so did others. I was also able to communicate what was going on and that I had no control over the noises I was making. My noises were a lot subtler too. Since, to me, my tics sounded like a hiccup, that is what they were, and that's how I responded to them and, thus, how other people responded to them. You can't control hiccups, and they are easily excused by other people. So my noises were permitted.

As I got older, the noises were not possible to pass off as a simple hiccup, but that is still how I saw them. I was able to communicate with others that I had no control over my noises and I had no idea what was going on, but I still didn't have an explanation for them.

But then I was diagnosed.

I feel like my identity has shifted since my diagnosis and since I started studying TS in depth. Before I learned about TS, I thought I knew who I was—thought I knew about my life with my "squeaks"—but then all of this new information came and changed everything. Now when I do anything, I know that I can look at my actions and determine whether they were caused by my TS, my OCD, or just my own conscious choices. Though sometimes it is hard to really tell.

Being diagnosed and learning more about TS has opened my eyes to much more than just my present actions though. Knowing what I know now, I realize that certain manifestations of my TS have been present for years. For example, since I was little, I have repeated funny lines in movies. In fact, people sometimes get really frustrated with how much I talk during movies. When I started reading more about TS, I learned about Echolalia (my type of TS—the repetition of words and phrases that an individual hears). Thinking back now, I realize that even in something like repeating movie lines, TS may have been in my life since I was young.

Once I learned I had TS, I stopped to look at my life and what that meant. That self-reflection led me to write a senior paper in college rather than doing an internship, and the subject of that paper has led to the writing of this book.

As I wrote that paper, I really dove into what TS was. I may have been diagnosed at 24, but, as I mentioned, I had been showing signs long before I even started making noises, as well as showing signs of OCD. Learning about TS was so incredibly liberating for me. I never would have realized how much a part of my life this was and how much it influenced me without my diagnosis. It gave an explanation for my quirks, and even if my quirks had never really been an obstacle I had to overcome, it was still helpful to understand myself better and have clarification about what was going on. Understanding myself and being informed about what I was experiencing was incredibly empowering. Who doesn't want that kind of freedom in their lives?

These reflections, as well as my progressing search for knowledge of my condition, continue to play with my ideas of who I think I am and what I do.

Lack of Understanding and Knowledge about Tourette Syndrome

Once an individual is diagnosed with TS (or even once a person starts exhibiting tics but hasn't yet been diagnosed), there are still many challenges in learning how to live with it. But on top of that, it can be a little challenging for other people to understand and adjust to it too.

For instance, one summer I was living at home with my parents. Before that summer, I hadn't been around my parents that much since I had graduated from high school (when my tics were beginning to emerge), and my tics had become much more developed since that time. As that summer showed me, and from what I've learned throughout the years since then, my tics can be a little hard on others.

My dad, and a lot of people actually, often had knee-jerk reactions about my tics, especially at first and when the tics were sudden and loud. Sometimes I used to see him getting really frustrated when my tics got particularly loud and high pitched. And it's understandable—they hurt his ears! Since that summer when I lived at home, my dad has gotten more used to my tics, but in the beginning, it was hard when he wasn't expecting them.

I can understand how some people would also have a hard time understanding the concept that I'm not in control of what I do. Because I've learned more about TS, I understand that my tics are completely involuntary. (They surprise me too!) But other people just don't know why I sometimes imitate sounds or randomly move my arm or whatever it is that Jess feels like doing that day. To an outsider, these things would probably just look strange. And it's hard that sometimes people just don't understand me or what I'm doing.

In every instance though, I try to give the other person the benefit of the doubt and to see things from the person's point of view. Over time, I've come to realize that when people don't know about TS, one small noise can really affect them. My tics can even scare people. In fact, they often do.

Just think: it would be scary to hear a person get the wind knocked out of him or her, especially if you don't see what happened or know what is going on. Just think of strangers passing by as I have a tic: they have no idea what is going on, even for the smaller (or bigger) noises that don't sound like anything scary.

This lack of understanding can be difficult. I think not feeling understood by others, or even by yourself, can make TS incredibly challenging on an emotional level.

Lack of Control of Your Body When You Have TS

One time, I went to a different church than I typically go to. I was sitting behind an entire row of girls, and during the most quiet part of the meeting, Jess decided not to be so quiet. In one quick motion, all of the girls jumped up at least a foot. It was difficult to stifle my giggle, but I managed to stay quiet. But then they all turned to glare at me, again in perfect unison, and I couldn't keep it in. I let out a few chuckles, which I'm sure didn't help their view of me. Luckily for me, I never saw them again.

Not really—I would have liked to explain myself and make new friends, but sometimes I don't always get to do that. They didn't understand that I couldn't control what I was doing, and that lack of physical control can be really challenging.

For instance, there are days when my physical tics can be incredibly active and painful—like on days when Jess gets upset. Jess is great! But on those days when she gets upset, it's just not pretty, and it never ends well for me.

One day at work, I got particularly frustrated on the phone with one of our contractors. As soon as I got off the phone, Jess went off, venting before I got the chance. Then, a shoulder tic started. The first one caught me so much by surprise and was so strong that my entire arm got thrown forward, missing my computer monitor by only an inch or two.

Let me just restate that for emphasis: Jess almost punched my work computer! She almost damaged company property!

And then she kept going! I was a little more prepared for the next tic and was able to keep most of my arm under control. But oh how that shoulder ticced! And this went on for the rest of the day—and it hurt every time.

I'm fairly certain that Jess threw my back out of alignment that day, because the next day I was very sore. Luckily, I had already scheduled a chiropractor appointment, which helped immensely. However, I certainly learned that Jess is not someone I want to upset. She doesn't get upset often, thankfully. She will chew out the occasional coworker who doesn't see her side of a discussion, but it's all in good fun. Jess likes to debate, especially since she tends to have the last word. She has plenty of those stories. (Only that one, however, almost damaged company property and sent me to a doctor!)

On another similar day, both of my shoulders and my back were moving way more than they should for a person who normally sits at a desk all day. The tics even went up into my neck a few times. They hurt so much that by the end of the day, I couldn't stand it anymore and asked a friend of mine to work out at least one massive knot I had in my back. As she worked, my right arm started turning red as I suddenly had so much more blood flowing through my veins. It worried me a little. Sometimes on days like that, I even need to go to a massage therapist to work out my sore muscles.

On top of my lack of control over my physical tics, I'm also discovering other things that are suddenly much harder to control than they used to be. For instance, the more organized I try to be, the more I see my OCD rear its ugly head, and I am getting really particular about details being in place.

Take my closet, for example: one time when I was moving, for the first time in my life, I color-coded my closet. As I was unpacking, I finished color-coding the shirts, and I was going to walk away and work on the next unpacking project. I didn't want to color-code my whole closet, but I couldn't just leave half of it undone.

I had to color-code the other half.

It was weird to have this struggle going on about something as silly as organizing a closet! I had so many other things I would rather have gotten done. But I couldn't stop myself. I couldn't leave until the task was done. I felt like I didn't have a choice—I had to do it. And that feeling of lack of control, not feeling like I was able to make my own decision and instead being compelled to do something that I just couldn't control, was so frustrating.

I'm not sure that people without TS or OCD, or any other quirk that prevents you from having complete control over your body, know exactly how terrible that kind of situation can feel—how terrifying and frustrating it is to understand on a rational level that you don't need to do something, like color-coding your closet, but feeling like you have to do it anyway.

The most distressing part I've noticed about my TS though comes from something I read in Disconnected Kids: The Groundbreaking Brain Balance Program for Children with Autism, ADHD, Dyslexia, and Other Neurological Disorders by Dr. Robert Melillo (2010). The book talks about how one half of the brain develops faster than the other half. According to Dr. Melillo, this also affects the development of our emotions. This little detail really stuck with me because I hate emotions.

I hate crying with a passion, and for the most part, I have detached myself from my emotions, because once I feel one emotion, I can't control anything that I'm feeling and everything hits at once and it's completely overwhelming. I can't handle emotions; that's why I shut them off.

When things are hard, I cry, but I hate crying so then I get angry, and then the logic tries to take over and say, "It's ok. You need to cry and this makes sense." and thus starts an ugly spiral of negative emotions and arguments inside my head that go back and forth trying to figure everything out until I get so exhausted that nothing makes sense anymore.

That's when I get to a snapping point.

I try to keep that in check, but sometimes it's a real struggle. In fact, I could see how when you're dealing with so many emotions, especially on top of uncontrollable physical and vocal tics and anxious tendencies, you could even become violent because that's the only way to get out and escape from your own mind.

Personally, I have had urges to smash glass, tear books, kick, scream, hit, and so on. I'll be the first one to admit: it's not a pretty picture. (See what I mean that you don't want to make Jess mad?) Keeping emotions all bottled up doesn't really help matters much. I don't know what to do with it all.

These are definitely some of the downsides of having Tourette's.

Social Difficulties: Cues and Symbols

In addition to the other struggles we've discussed in this chapter, one more common struggle for those with TS is difficulty understanding social cues and symbols. However, before we can really discuss not understanding social cues, it's important for us to fully understand what social cues are themselves. So let's talk about that first.

Social cues are nothing more than symbols we use to communicate with other people. Kenneth Burke, an American philosopher and theorist, wrote a wonderful definition of man that helps us see how symbols and communication are connected. He defined man as a "symbol-using (symbol-making, symbol-misusing) animal" (Burke 2012). As Burke shows in this definition, everything we do involves symbols, whether or not we like to admit it.

Who is to say that a random bunch of sounds (verbal words) means the same thing as a random bunch of squiggles on a piece paper (written words)? Words are symbols used to facilitate understanding, and we use and interpret these symbols on a constant basis. Even the tone of voice used can show whether a person is using sarcasm or is completely sincere. And consider body language as well—body language is yet another way in which we interpret certain actions to mean different things. For instance, you know what I'm thinking if I am rolling my eyes. Eye rolling, as well as other verbal and nonverbal cues, is a symbol we interpret, and from that symbol we create understanding.

But everyone is raised with different experiences interpreting symbols, so with all of this individual interpretation, it's easy to see how miscommunication takes place. In fact, it's interesting to me how many conflicts arise because of a simple miscommunication. Sometimes miscommunications may be due to being raised in different geographic locations. For example, in North America, if I were to point at something with my hand or finger, that's no big deal. However, in many Asian countries, that same gesture is considered to be rude.

The interpretation of symbols may vary even within the United States. I grew up in Nevada, and some of the phrases we use are not used in South Carolina, where my dad's family comes from, and vice versa. The first time I heard the phrase "farsee," for instance, I had no idea what it was. (Eventually I learned that "farsee" is a term used for giving directions and it means going as far as you can see. ("They live about three farsees that way.") Or consider the ever-present battle: pop or soda? The lack of understanding of symbols, or of having different understandings of symbols, can create all sorts of awkward situations. This makes it hard to coordinate with other people at times.

When you have a quirk like TS, sometimes symbols are even more difficult to understand. For instance, sometimes I just flat-out don't get sarcasm, or I don't understand when people use subtext and don't really say what they mean. Or sometimes it's just hard for me to completely follow a conversation, especially when that conversation takes a turn or doesn't head where I'm expecting it to. I just think more literally, and so I sometimes misunderstand when other people aren't communicating that way and are using symbols differently than I do.

I have one friend who salvaged one of my friendships with his ability to understand the symbols going on around us (when I wasn't fully able to). I was at a group gathering at someone's house. We had been talking about pet peeves, and Jess sounded an awful lot like one person's pet peeve. At one point, Jess let out a loud squeal, and the girl became (understandably) upset because she thought I was making the noise on purpose. As I sometimes don't even notice when I make noises, or maybe because I'm so used to them, I didn't really understand why the girl was so upset. The symbols being exchanged between me and this person just weren't being understood by both of us. Until people realize that my tics are tics, sometimes they think I'm simply communicating, and in this situation, the girl was offended by my communication. Luckily, a mutual friend of ours stepped in and explained everything, essentially saving both me and the girl embarrassment and further misunderstanding.

In that exchange, I just wasn't connecting the symbols and didn't understand fully what was going on and, therefore, I wasn't able to defend myself. Once my friend explained the situation though, the girl apologized profusely.

Our mutual friend, and his ability to help us communicate and interpret symbols, saved that conversation and allowed me and the girl to actually develop a strong friendship moving forward.

How to Be the Author of Your Life Story

Now that we have a solid foundation in understanding TS and the struggles that sometimes come with it, let's talk about how we can embrace our lives to the fullest, despite those struggles. In this chapter, I'll discuss numerous tips and suggestions on how to address common TS struggles and, ultimately, tell the story of your life as you want it to be written.

Improve Communication

In the last chapter, we talked about social cues and symbols and how those affect how we interact with others. You may have noticed that many of the struggles around TS are simply about communication: we have to be able to communicate effectively to get a proper diagnosis and we have to communicate with others about what we're going through so they can better understand us. And, as we discussed, it's challenging when we don't have control over how we communicate. Further, it's difficult when we do have control over our communication but we don't understand the symbols others are using to communicate with us.

It's all about communication.

Right now, improving your communication skills might sound like a lofty goal. But take it from someone who's lived with

TS for quite a few years now: you can improve your communication with a couple simple tips. So, let's talk about them.

Observe and read. A lot.

As a child, I spent a lot of time reading. And when I say "a lot," I mean that my parents were concerned with how much I was reading, and eventually I was grounded from books for an entire summer! Although I gained a lot from reading so much, looking back, I realize that I also probably lost a lot as well. I can see where reading so much may have caused a disconnect in my brain.

Maybe my parents subconsciously recognized that and were hoping that by taking a little break from reading, I would get out and play more. I see the value in what my parents were trying to accomplish with this "grounding," but, honestly, I think, overall, reading was incredibly beneficial for me and for my TS, even if I didn't yet know that I had TS.

Allow me to explain. When I was younger, I had a terrible social life, but it was always something that I wanted to improve. I wanted to have friends and to be social, so I set out to learn all that I could about people. Believe it or not, I actually learned a lot about human nature from the fiction books I read as a child, and I became an observer in social situations. I think this was beneficial to me because I got an inside look at how people thought and acted and the connection between the two. I watched people and learned a lot there as well. This was all as I was very young, before I even started to make vocal noises.

I guess there's some truth to my belief that I learned a lot through observation: one researcher, Albert Bandura, studied the effects of observation on our behavior (Fryling, Johnston, and Hayes, 2011). Three other researchers did some follow-up on his findings. In their 2011 article "Understanding Observational Learning: An Interbehavioral Approach" in The Analysis of Verbal Behavior, authors Mitch J Fryling, Cristin Johnston, and Linda J Hayes describe Bandura's findings, saying "Behavior change can and does occur through observation, even when such observation is incidental, occurring in the context of other activities. While this finding seems rather simple, it has significant implications for how we conceptualize learning."

Basically, whether we mean to or not, we are constantly learning from others. We see things that we either do or don't want to repeat and keep a mental log of these things. When similar situations come into our lives, we remember what we saw/heard before and it affects how we respond to these situations.

While the authors recognized that Bandura's studies were not perfect, they did agree with the overall idea of how much simple observation affects how we act. As I have found out in my own personal experience, observation has been incredibly helpful in learning how to interact in social situations.

As I studied human behavior, both through reading and personal observation, I learned how people interact. It was helpful to me to hear from various characters what they expected from a typical social interaction and to also hear about their reactions when they were in atypical social situations.

I got lost in these books, in learning about different worlds and characters and situations. And I think, overall, I was able to use the critical thinking and observation skills that I learned by reading those books to better observe human behavior in real life and, thus, apply those observations in my own life.

So although I think it's essential to have balance, I'd highly recommend taking the time to read, read, and read more and to become a private investigator of human interactions in everyday life.

Always consider context!

In all social interactions, it's essential to consider the context in which things are said. You know how we discussed symbols earlier? Well, symbols require context to be understood.

You have to speak the local language in order to understand conversations going on around you. You have to be able to read to know what the words in this sentence mean when they're all placed together like this. Better yet, you have to read an entire paragraph, or paper, or book, in order to fully get the context of a single sentence. If you pull a single sentence from this book, you may infer something very different from what that sentence was intended to mean. This puts everyone on the same page and is called coordination.

This is why we feel the need to investigate interruptions in conversations, and really, in general. Now, if you thought difficulties in coordination were awkward, wait until you experience interruption! New, random symbols are constantly tossed into conversation, and no one has any idea what is going on. In fact, sometimes an interruption will stop a conversation all together.

For instance, say you're chatting with a friend, and someone screams. (Now there's an interruption!) During that type of situation, we tend to drop our flow of symbols in order to investigate the interruption and where it is coming from. The scream may have come from a person screaming in fear while walking through a haunted house, a person screaming in physical pain because of an accident, a person screaming in delight when passing a test or being accepted to college, or a myriad of other causes. See how the same symbol can bring so many emotions to the surface? Fear, joy, anger, and sorrow are all possible because of an interruption.

The point is, however, that interruptions are new symbols we suddenly and unexpectedly have to deal with.

Only the source of an interruption will help us fully understand what the symbol is and what it means. This is where having TS becomes the highlight of my life and is oh so much fun! Sometimes, I might be the source of the scream—I can't help it; they just pop out sometimes. In those situations, no one knows what is going on until I let them in on my secret. I gasp, I scream, I make an assortment of animal noises without warning, and most people make assumptions about what I'm doing, without context.

This means that I get to provide them with the context. And this means that I control the situation. Let me repeat that for you in case you missed it... I. Have. Control. I may not be able to control my body or my noises all of the time, but I control the story others hear and how things move forward from this point. I think this is an even greater power than having the control I lack with TS.

I love to watch the reactions of people the first time they experience my TS, especially if a particular noise falls in line with the context. A joyous shout from me may come directly after someone shares good news. It entertains me how many people will cheer along after my Tourette's decides to make such a timely appearance

In fact, the timing of my TS is so often well-placed that sometimes people don't believe I even have it! Jess is my favorite because during the times when I do have tics that seem out of context with a social situation, she starts a lot of conversations. Like I mentioned before, people have a curiosity to find out what interruptions are. We have a driving need to understand the world around us. The situations where Jess interrupts things are almost always awkward, but I love them, and I am in control of the situation. I revel in the awkwardness. Sometimes I feel like a jerk watching the confusion on someone's face, or on occasion, even fear, at what noises Jess is making, and all I can do is laugh.

For example, when I first met my friend Jeff, the subject of TS came up. We chatted for a good fifteen minutes about it, with him asking questions (and me feeling all sorts of intelligent that I could explain so much about it—"Why yes. Yes, I do have TS, and I've read loads about it. Does that make me an expert? Well, I don't want to brag, but..."). (Just kidding.) I even told him I had TS, so he knew about it. The conversation drifted, as most conversations do, but it was still only a good way into the conversation that Jess decided to make an appearance. It was a long, almost chatty, noise and it was right in his face. I watched him cower back the longer it went on. My friend, having never experienced Jess, had no idea what was happening. Even knowing that I had TS, he hadn't connected the two ideas. To him, Jess's noises were an interruption that needed explanation.

At first, these types of situations caught me off guard. Jess makes an appearance where and when she chooses, not me. Sometimes I don't even notice that she has popped up. For instance, once, Jess made two or three appearances in a group setting, and I hadn't thought to explain because I hadn't really noticed. All of a sudden, I was yelled at by a guy playing the piano to "stop it!" Luckily, I have awesome friends who jump to my defense, in this case yelling right back, "She can't stop it!" The piano player, again, not understanding fully what was going on, kept yelling, "What? Does she have Tourette's or something?"

Needless to say, he was quite embarrassed to learn that I did, indeed, have TS, and he wrote me a song as an apology.

As these stories show, communication is all about context. When I sometimes struggle to understand a situation, it's become invaluable for me to stop and think about the context in which something is said or the context in which an interruption takes place. Considering context has helped me exponentially in communicating and interacting with others, and it can help you too.

You choose which stories to believe.

We've talked a little about stories and context and how different people interpret symbols and situations differently. When you're wanting to take control of your life, especially when you have TS, I've learned that it's important to recognize that you can decide which stories are true for you.

The way that you decide to treat TS, or any other neurological quirk for that matter, depends on which story you believe about what causes it. Furthermore, if you go to a doctor and the doctor prescribes you a certain medication, that doctor is working from the stories that he or she believes, and you have a choice in deciding whether you also believe that same medical story.

Now, it's important for me to state here that, obviously, doctors are trained medical professionals, so I think it's important to give consideration to a professional medical opinion. But, as we've discussed, there's no agreed upon explanation for the causes of TS or agreed upon course of treatment. So, if you're considering your treatment options for TS, keep in mind that you get to decide what's right for you and which stories to believe.

For example, a doctor may recommend medication to help placate tics. I know this is not a path I want to pursue. I like my tics and I would miss Jess horribly if she disappeared. I do not want to deal with side effects, especially when there is no guarantee for how well the medication will work. You may find a book with more natural "cures." These natural "cures" work for some but don't work for others. Be open and willing to try new things—you might be surprised what will work, but know your own limitations as well.

This idea of choosing which stories to believe also relates to the stories that other people tell you, whether it's about yourself, or about the wider world, in general. Think back to that story I mentioned about the girls in front of me at church. When they got upset that I made noises, and they didn't know that I had TS, they glared at me. Their interpretation of the story of me making noises: I'm rude. My interpretation of the story: I have TS, and I can't help the sounds that I make, and I know I'm not rude. I could've taken their interpretation of the situation as being true, but I decided instead to believe my own story—that I have TS and those sounds that I make are completely normal. I have no need to feel ashamed of what I do.

Just think how differently I would've felt if I'd decided to believe that I was rude, based on those girls' stories. I would've left church feeling bad about myself and probably feeling misunderstood. But instead, I decided to just laugh at the situation (and to laugh at the girls' reaction), knowing that the girls just didn't have all the facts.

But it's not just other people who tell us stories about us. Throughout the years, we also tell ourselves stories about who we are and what we're capable of. Sometimes these stories may be true, but sometimes they aren't. When we recognize that we don't have to passively accept these stories as facts, we start to empower ourselves to create our own stories and choose what to believe.

When you sometimes feel like you don't have control of your life, whether it's because of TS or whatever life throws at you, it's important to know that we still have control over our own story.

Become a Trickster

Are you ready for another secret? Let's talk a little bit about Tricksters. German philosopher Georg Wilhelm Friedrich Hegel claims that "only the whole is true" (Spencer and Andrzej 1996). A statement is not fully true until we acknowledge its opposite. Who we are is shaped by what we are not. For those with TS, we are not "normal"; we are Tricksters. We have the capability to carry both ends of that spectrum (what we are and what we are not). We have an added characteristic used to help define what we are and what we are not. That can be taken in very different ways, as good or as bad. But that fact, in itself, gives us power and can help us take control of our lives.

So what is a Trickster?

Michael Webster, a professor of English at Grand Valley State University, gives a great definition of a Trickster in his course notes for a World Mythology course offered at the university

> A Trickster is a mischievous or roguish figure in myth or folklore who typically makes up for physical weakness with cunning and subversive humor. The Trickster alternates between cleverness and stupidity, kindness and cruelty, deceiver and deceived, breaker of taboos and creator of culture. (2005)

As Webster describes, Tricksters are trouble makers, but somehow things are able to fall into place for them. There are some positive and some negative results from the acts of the Trickster, and the views of the individual Trickster himself or herself determine whether the acts are good or bad. He creates his own story. Not only his own story, but the stories around him that create the culture as well.

A modern example of a Trickster would be Captain Jack Sparrow, played by Johnny Depp in the movie series Pirates of the Caribbean (2003–2011). Sometimes it's hard to tell whose side Captain Sparrow is on. He is hard to trust, but he always manages to follow through with both sides on all his deals. Things may not always go his way, but he still manages to come out on top of whatever game he is playing at the time. He has moments of great kindness and moments where he appears impossibly cruel. He speaks of things that should not be spoken of, has an insatiable curiosity, and loves to break the rules. He is a trickster to a T!

In The Social Life of Narrative: Marshall Islands, author Phillip McArthur also talks about Tricksters. "[T]he struggle for identity in a postmodern world is much like a trickster," he says; "Self-reflexivity is at times ambivalent and at other times brilliantly creative" (McArthur 1995, 85). He continues to explain that Tricksters break rules of society according to their whims and desires. And when Tricksters break the rules, everyone is forced to look at the rules of society. Tricksters bring the rules into question, and people with TS, well—let's just say that we're really good at breaking society's rules, surprising people, and making them ask questions that they may not otherwise ask.

Now that we've talked about how TS plays with an individual's identity, let's also talk about how the identity can play with TS. A Trickster in the form of identity will use events and twist them to the Trickster's advantage. I have done this numerous times, as have my friends. Knowing that I have Tourette Syndrome allows them to play with the interruptions and create new meanings.

For example, once, a boyfriend and I were at a social dinner, and he had gotten up to take our plates to the garbage. When he went across the room to throw the plates away so we could leave, he was soon distracted by a conversation. So when Jess made a loud squeal that echoed through the room, I heard him yell back to me, "Coming!" He used the interruption to break away from the conversation, and we were able to leave the dinner. He became the Trickster, manipulating the circumstances to his advantage and bringing a number of laughs with it.

The point remains that people with TS, or any other quirks, are different from most other people. We do something that few others do, and we cannot control it. However, that does not mean we have no control. We can control the situation once a tic has appeared, and we are able to guide the interpretation of a situation based on how we handle it.

The gap between "normal" and "different" can be very wide if taken to the idea of being, or existing. The spectrum of human behavior is so large that it is next to impossible to define "normal." People are all so very different that we have to narrow down our own view in order to see what is different. We would have to look at a specific group in order to see who really stands out. Change the group, and you change "normal." The difference allows for the presence of a Trickster in the forming of the identity. The Trickster would be someone who would jump in between groups, making the groups question the idea of "normal."

The individual who knows and understands what is going on (the person with TS) has the upper hand in manipulating a situation. Others who do not understand are left trying to figure out what happened, giving the individual with TS a chance to explain. The individual's story then becomes the reality, rather than whatever interpretation the other people may have come up with on their own. "Normal," then, becomes whatever the Trickster determines is normal.

Don't be afraid to go against the grain.

Simply put: Tricksters go against the grain. So if you want to be a Trickster and have more control over social situations, sometimes you have to take the road less traveled.

I once read a story of a girl who lost her leg. It had to be amputated in order to save her life. Similar to those with TS, she got a lot of attention. This girl told the story of a little boy who was staring at her leg. He was even bold enough to ask what had happened.

Acting like a true Trickster, the girl leaned in and whispered to the boy that he shouldn't tell anyone, but she is actually a transformer.

I loved the example of this brave girl and what she did to her story. She could have told a tragic tale of woe about how she lost her leg. But instead of surrendering to her story and letting the sadness get her down, she created an inspiring tale that brought a bit of magic into the life of at least one little boy. And I'm sure there are many more stories like this.

This story actually relates to my favorite part of having TS: being around little children and seeing their reactions to my tics. I wish all adults could be more like children, as this is where some of my greatest moments come from. With any luck, the best teaching moments for you will come from these kinds of situations as well.

The reason it's so great to have Tourette's and interact with children is that children have no idea what is acceptable in culture; they have no idea of what is "normal" yet. They are young and are still learning the rules of the social game. This is why they are so open to something that can be so different. However, even at that young age, we can see how culture is starting to shape them.

One poignant example is in the movie 42: The Jackie Robinson Story about the life of Jackie Robinson (2013). There is one scene that is forever etched into my memory: a little boy is at a baseball game and he is so excited to be there. When Jackie comes onto the field, the little boy watches his father scream racial slurs and terms of hatred at the baseball player. For a moment, the boy is torn between his admiration of the game and those who play, and the example of his beloved father. The boy then begins to scream racial slurs as well, influenced by those around him, even though he didn't fully understand what was going on (42: The Jackie Robinson Story 2013).

Or consider a happier example, when I was in university, I had some friends who lived with their family, and their extended family often visited. One member of the extended family was a cute little three-year-old named Tipa. Tipa loved all the attention he got from the college kids as we gathered at his home. At one point, as he was being his cute little self, Jess jumped out screaming!

Tipa jumped and turned around with big eyes full of fear that he had done something wrong. My friends all knew what was going on, so they laughed at the cute and terrified expression on his face. Once he realized he was not in trouble and he saw our laughter, he figured I was playing some kind of trick on him, and he slapped me! (I chose to take it as a sign of affection as he was smiling when he did.)

Another three-year-old had a slightly different reaction. Every time Jess showed up, he would smile at me and, on occasion, he would mimic Jess's noises. As Jess tends to speak out more when someone is having a conversation with her, the two would go back and forth several times.

What I loved about these experiences of mine was the opportunity to teach that people are different, and even if you don't understand it, you can really have a good time when things don't turn out the way you expect them to. Kids get that! They just go with the flow and have a good time because they don't have any context for how things "should" be. Because of this lack of expectation of "normal," children don't try to alter and control situations (like we often do as adults) to make things the way they "should" be.

I think as adults we sometimes lose that childlike ability to respond to situations without judgment about what we were taught is socially acceptable. As we grow older, we tend to learn which rules work best for us, and we become passionate about those rules. Now remember, these rules are essentially man-made, but they become stricter and more rigid as we follow them longer and longer. I'm not saying rigidity is a bad thing, but it does make life less playful. This can vary by person.

When I meet new people, I get so many different reactions and accusations about my tics. Instead of asking what's going on or taking these interruptions in stride, like children often do, adults are sometimes afraid to ask about what is going on, thinking that it's rude to ask, and often stare or else they sometimes assume the worst (e.g., that I'm being rude or seeking attention).

Before I was diagnosed, I would always get asked where I was hiding the mouse or squeaky toy. I heard that one so many times that it wasn't funny anymore. Another interesting response: my uncle used to ask me if I ever drank oil. I replied that I hadn't, and I asked why he suggested that I'd do such a thing. "Well," he figured, "It helps squeaky doors, so maybe it would help you!"

To this day, at one party a person may yell at me when I have a tic, and at another party someone else will have a completely different reaction. I think the most comical (and maybe my favorite) reaction I ever got was at one particular birthday party. There was a young man there who looked at me when I made a noise and asked, "Is that your mating call? 'Cause it's working!"

Although at some point we learn the rules of the game (i.e., what is "normal"), when we learn those rules, we can also learn how to bend and play with them. For instance, some of my other most memorable experiences are with my friends who talk back to Jess and treat her as her own person, playing upon societal rules. In fact, it is easiest to be around my friends when Jess decides to show up.

My grandmother also treats Jess as another one of her own grandchildren, and I love the extra hugs I get as she embraces Jess and thanks her for showing up after I have already gotten my hugs! As my friends and family often show me, sometimes the best things happen when people aren't afraid to play with the rules and go against the "normal" grain.

So, let's talk about you.

So let's get real here: let's talk about strengths and weaknesses.

I know, I know—you think you've heard this before: "I need to know what I'm good at and what I need to work on in order to be the best version of myself!"

Well, yes—actually that's true. But I'm not just going to say that.

We're not just going to talk about our weaknesses so we can move past them and our strengths so we can fully use them but rather talk about how your weaknesses ARE your strengths if you know how to use them. We tend to undervalue ourselves and under-utilize the character traits we have. They can sometimes be seen as "negative" and society sometimes tells us that you need to get rid of them, but I suggest that weaknesses are just strengths that we are using wrong. For example, anger is an important emotion, and we feel it for a reason, but that doesn't mean we should go around having temper tantrums. Anger needs to be controlled to a degree to give it the most strength.

Work on your weaknesses and celebrate your strengths

While you may be eager to jump right in and get rid of negative qualities that hold you back, part of the process of progression and improvement is to take inventory of your qualities and really assess which qualities are helping you be your best and which qualities may need some work. Knowing how to use the traits you possess is what makes you strong. It is what makes you comfortable with yourself and gives you confidence.

Now, don't get me wrong, I'm not saying that this means you should just completely get rid of the so-called "bad" traits all together. Consider the trait of stubbornness: it's not something we need to eradicate, just refine. Being stubborn can be a good thing. It's good to stick to things without being swayed by popular opinion. This is usually called tenacity. Same trait, different uses. I'm saying that it's important to use your qualities—the good qualities and the ones you'd rather work on—to your advantage and to harness the traits to work for you, not against you.

For me, part of discovering the areas I struggled in was finding new concepts I wanted to explore. For example, I mentioned earlier that I used to have a terrible social life, but it was something that I wanted to improve. I wanted to have friends and be social, so I set out to learn all I could about people, and the best way I could learn about human nature was to read (a lot!) and become an avid observer in social situations.

Then, once I started making noises, I suddenly had a lot more attention than I was used to having just watching people. The time for observing was past, and it was now time to jump in and start putting to practice the things I had learned about people and interacting. I still wasn't very good at it though. As I got into college, I started out with different majors, but none were as satisfying as what I graduated in. My degree is essentially in the sociology field with an emphasis in communications. I was still studying how people interact and communicate with one another.

In the end, I decided that instead of being defined by the things I wanted to work on, I would recognize and acknowledge my weaknesses and then meet them head on. By using my weakness, such as my social skills, as an opportunity for learning, I was able to gradually build my social skills and, ultimately, make a career out of them.

And other people do this same thing every day—even people with TS or other quirks—in fact, especially those people with TS or other quirks.

Take my friend Emma, for instance. When Emma was only five, she was already showing signs of OCD and TS. She got in trouble for being a distraction in class and had other similar experiences. So, as a release for her tics, Emma eventually became a drummer. She was always banging on things anyway, so she figured she would put the habit to good use (Personal interview with Emma Hardy 2012).

Having TS has shaped her life so much that without it, she would be a completely different person. Without this one trait (TS), she would not have thought of becoming a drummer. The choices she made and who she became would have been a completely different person. She once told me, "I'm a potato. Without my Tourette Syndrome, I wouldn't be who I am. I don't know if I would still be a drummer or in theatre tech. I would be a completely different person. I would feel blank without it" (Personal interview with Emma Hardy 2012).

And that's what I admire about Emma: how she was able to take negative experiences from her childhood and turn them into something beautiful.

In *Don't Think about Monkeys: Extraordinary Stories by People with Tourette Syndrome* Mitch Vitiello tells a similar story. He explained having "migraine headaches from moving my head so much" (Seligman and Hilkevich 1992,11). He recounted stories of walking home when his shoulder would suddenly jerk up so violently that it hit his ear or of being unable to hold a pencil from all the twitching. His entire body would twitch and jerk at intervals.

Mitch had a family that was always loving and supportive, giving him the counsel that he needed in order to feel comfortable with who he was, even when he was not. It was his dad who gave the advice that changed Mitch's personal ideas, helped him accept what was happening, and live the life that he wanted. In fact, Mitch's symptoms even decreased after taking his dad's advice. His father told Mitch that he had to learn to deal with it and that "if you act like it bothers you, it would bother other people. Act like it is nothing and they will forget about it" (Seligman and Hilkevich 1992, 12).

Another story went beyond the idea of just feeling comfortable with TS, to an ability to "harness the enormous energy of Tourette Syndrome and control it like a high pressure fire hose" (Seligman and Hilkevich 1992). David Aldridge developed motor tics that made him drum his fingers and bang on various objects. These were tics found alongside his blinking, neck and head movements, and vocal tics. He found at a young age that drumming, when focused in music classes and on drum sets, gave him "permission to explode" (Seligman and Hilkevich 1992).

Combined with the rhythms he could hear in his head, the drumming allowed him to become a "Rhythm Man" (Seligman and Hilkevich 1992, 174–175). Drumming became a form of therapy where David could release the anger, hurt, and frustrations he felt from being teased about his TS at school. All of the practice of drumming on things paid off and Aldridge became a musician. As a musician, his TS symptoms were not only tolerated but "met with applause" (Seligman and Hilkevich 1992, 177).

As these stories show, it is possible to not only live with your struggles but to embrace the areas that you want to improve and use them to transform your life.

In my own life, for example, I try to channel certain facets of my OCD into my professional work. Even the light touch of OCD that I have I know I can use to my advantage. Having an attention to detail is something most work places look for, and it is encouraged. When interviewing for a job, or even when I'm collaborating with my coworkers, I am sure to let them know that I will be able to get details taken care of and I'll ensure that tasks are completed from beginning to end.

Personally, I know that's true because I always have this nagging in the back of my mind if something isn't finished. My OCD simply needs a sense of completion. I can't tell you how much this has helped me in my work situations.

I use work as my outlet. I let my OCD go absolutely crazy while I am at work, making sure everything has that sense of completion and organization. Even if the way I work looks like chaos to someone else, my chaos has a system.

And while details and specifics may vary from person to person, I am not the only one in need of an outlet. We all need to have an environment where we are able to let our oddities run rampant.

For me, my OCD is best suited at for any kind of task that requires attention to detail and great organizational skills. My friend Emma became a drummer as an outlet for her tics and twitches. Another person from my hometown is autistic and is an absolute genius when it comes to computers and software. He was hired by a company that allows him to utilize his genius. Sure, he needs someone to remind him to take a shower in the mornings and go through his morning routine, but once he gets to work, they give him his own little room with all the tools he needs to do his job. They understand how his mind works, leave him to it, and he does a great job.

Sometimes I get frustrated with the way the autism spectrum is viewed. People are so focused on what we can't do that they don't realize what we can. Sometimes people don't realize how intuitive people on the autism spectrum are. We may think differently than most people, but isn't that supposed to be a good thing? Look at any great person in history. Da Vinci certainly thought differently than anyone else in his time. Look at the genius who was so far ahead of his time—Tesla was thought to be crazy. Think about how people must have looked at the Wright brothers when they said, "We're going to build a machine that can fly!" What it comes down to is this: we live in a world that needs that "spark of madness," as actor Robin Williams once said, in order to move forward. We need people who think unlike others and can create new systems and programs, and even new ways of thinking, or we stop growing and moving forward. To have such incredibly intelligent people (and by this statement, I mean you!) among us is such a gift to humanity.

Everyone will use their strengths and their weaknesses differently, but that fact in itself—the fact that we're all so different—is powerful. There is strength in the differences, in the traits that maybe right now you think are disadvantages or weaknesses.

TS is what makes me different. It also unites me to people I would have otherwise never met. I consider this my super power. What is yours? What makes you special, unique, and different? Different is good, I promise. Whatever it is, it will be your springboard into life's adventures.

Up to this point, I thought I had no passion and that I was incapable of having passion for anything. But understanding myself gave me drive and direction. It gave me validation that I am who I am, and my weird ideas and habits aren't that uncommon. Understanding myself allowed me to redefine "normal."

The things I do, like screaming in the middle of a meeting at work, are completely normal. Once everyone at work is filled in on what is going on, no one else even bats an eye when it happens. Unless the timing is really good and it gives us a chance to laugh! The more we learn about the disruption of the symbols we hold so dear, we can adopt new symbols and move forward with a greater understanding of ourselves and of the world around us.

At this point, I want to make it clear that I'm not saying that having TS isn't hard. As much as I love my vocal tics, Jess has sent me to the chiropractor. I have a physical tic that makes my right shoulder jerk forward. Sometimes it's small, just like a shudder, and people ask if I am cold all the time. Other times, it can jerk forward so suddenly I almost punch my computer at work. That would not have ended well and scared me a bit, despite my laughing about it later. I have come pretty close to giving myself whiplash and throwing off the entire alignment of my spine. It can be very painful when she jerks that hard.

Celebrate Your Quirks and Own Your Weirdness

Ok, so the title of this section may bring a questioning look to your face, but just hear me out. Part of living with TS is accepting the fact that TS is something you can't control. Really, what it all comes down to is this: don't fight it; own it.

<u>Let it go, let it go! Can't hold it back anymore! (i.e., Let go of the things you can't control.)</u>

After my tics started changing in high school, I remember how sometimes I used to worry about them. Although I was ok with them, I was a little concerned about the fact that my parents were concerned about me. And of course there was the fact that no one really knew why I was making random sounds…That was a little distressing.

But I don't only remember the times that I worried about my TS. I also remember the specific day when I decided to stop worrying about it.

It was in May 2007. At that point, I hadn't yet been diagnosed with TS, so I wasn't exactly sure what was going on, but I knew my tics had been evolving and changing, and I had started to notice that they were becoming more frequent. This particular day in May was no exception to that.

I was going to the temple for the first time, and I had very little idea of what to expect. I lay in bed the night before, tossing and turning, picturing what it would be like to go to the temple. I'd prepared myself for this big day, but all I knew for sure was that I was making covenants and promises to God. The sense of mystery and anticipation had me pacing back and forth after breakfast, made me jittery as if I'd had one too many cups of coffee (which I don't even drink), and interested Jess so much that she was making noises about every five minutes or so as my mom and I drove around Las Vegas running errands beforehand. In fact, I can't think of any time since then that my tics have been that active!

However, once I stepped inside the temple, something changed. I don't know what it was, but suddenly, I went quiet. The tics had stopped.

Trips to the temple usually take about two hours or less, but the first time through, I think it takes about four or five hours with everything that is going on. And NOT ONCE in those four or five hours did Jess make an appearance.

That's not the end of the story though! It's one thing for tics to come and to go—maybe I was just done for the day and I wouldn't have any more tics the rest of the evening…

But that wasn't the case. What stands out most to me about that day is the dinner I had with my family after our visit to the temple. Everyone who had joined me in the temple that day came to dinner with us at Olive Garden. (I love Italian food!) Almost as soon as we got our seats, I squeaked. We all had a good chuckle at the confused waiter.

And the squeaks kept coming.

And coming.

And before we knew it, they were coming every five minutes like they had before I stepped into the temple.

That was the point where I quit worrying about my tics. After that day, all worry and concern on my part stopped. My line of thinking went something along the lines of, "Clearly our

Heavenly Father loves and respects these sacred places. If He cared enough to silence my noises for so long so I could focus on what was going on around me, He would surely do it again if there was ever a need for it. He knows me. He knows what these noises are, and He has it under control."

I understand that not everyone will have the same religious beliefs that I do. That's ok. No matter what your belief system may be, I would encourage a belief in the idea that there are reasons for everything. I happen to believe in a loving God who knows me personally and what I need in my life. I think that idea rings true no matter what your beliefs. I don't believe that who we are and the qualities and gifts we are born with are any kind of accident. I don't believe in accidents. (Except maybe knocking over a glass of water.)

I have never worried about my tics since then. I have been free to laugh and enjoy them without any reservation. That simple act of letting go of my worry and of trying to control my tics has made such an impact in my life. I know it's hard sometimes to not have control of your body and to know that there's no agreed-upon medical explanation for what you're going through. But I know too that it's pointless to worry about something that you have no control over. What's the point in wasting your life trying to change something that you can't, when, instead, you could be celebrating who you are?

This leads us to my next suggestion…

Celebrate your quirks instead of hiding them.

The more I write about Jess and her personality, the more I realize how much like an individual she really is. I have about as much control over what Jess does as I'd have over what any other person does, in general (that is to say: not much…ok, let's be real: no control; Jess has a mind of her own!). But once I decided to let go and accept the fact that Jess refuses to listen to me (thanks, Jess), I have become ever so much closer to her and I have come to better understand her and her personality. And I have to say: Jess is pretty cool.

This journey of getting to know Jess, and, thus, myself, reminds me of a memory from elementary school. Once a week we had a music class, and the teacher always started class off with a positive affirmation. It was always the same one and was several lines long. But I just remember one line: "I'm my own best friend and my own worst enemy."

I feel like Jess has helped me understand this phrase on a completely new level. There are times when I may be absolutely infuriated with Jess. Like I mentioned (multiple times in this book because it's not just true, it's so true), sometimes it isn't easy not being in control of your own body and actions. But, on the other hand, sometimes it can be the funniest thing in the world. Jess can be my biggest trial and my biggest blessing all at the same time. She is talented like that I guess. Jess is just like the younger sibling you grew up fighting with, but you know she always has your back.

And just like you think you know your siblings and then they do something that surprises you, Jess often surprises me. Take her communication skills, for instance: Jess often has full conversations with people when they're willing to engage with her. I just have to laugh about these interactions and how drawn out the conversations are. I don't always notice how they start, but Jess does love her conversations with one of my coworkers. While I may not recall the exact phrasing of every conversation, they usually follow some pattern like this:

> Coworker: Can I get a little help over here?
> Jess: *unintelligible squeaking*
> Coworker: No, Jess, I need a team lead.
> Jess: *faster squeaking*
> Coworker: Don't sass me Jess...
> Jess: *who knows at this point...*

At which point we both crack up laughing. The conversations may vary, but Jess and my coworker have become good friends and keep each other on their toes. Jess finally has a friend who will sass her right back when she's feeling feisty, and my coworker has someone to keep her in line at work. I think this is a good arrangement.

There was another time at work where I just had to laugh at Jess and her sense of humor. It was Halloween and one of my coworkers dressed up as a scarecrow. When Jess saw her, Jess barked. (As I discussed in Chapter 1, I do a lot of animal sounds, but I don't often bark like a dog. Jess leans toward more exotic animals like peacocks. So the barking like a small dog is relatively new.) Also in good humor, my friend replied that that wasn't quite the scarecrow she was going for, but that Jess could be her Toto.

Jess got a little quiet for a while until another coworker asked what Jess was for Halloween. She then barked again. I think Jess liked the idea of being Toto for Halloween, and many of my vocal tics that day were barking. There were a few festive

Halloween noises tossed in as well. She threw a few ghost noises out, and an opera singer or two, but they were always creepy and dark and very fitting given the time of year.

I love how interactions and situations like this help me to celebrate my TS instead of having to hide it. I'm so glad that my coworkers, friends, and family are so accepting of my TS. They simply embrace who I am, and it makes it so much easier for me to do the same.

I'm glad I'm to the point where I celebrate my quirks (i.e., Jess and her outgoing personality) not just for my own emotional wellbeing though…I'm happy I can embrace my TS, because I'm not sure that Jess would keep quiet even if I wanted her to! In fact, sometimes Jess is like a bratty teenager—she likes the spotlight, and she'll tell you when she's got something on her mind, whether or not you want to hear it. Like the other day: my roommate was sharing a story and Jess interrupted her quite rudely.

I just can't stop her! So what's the point in trying? I may as well laugh about all the funny things she does and just move on!

Develop a Solid Support System

Humans are social creatures. Regardless of a person's age or background, relationships are a key component of human development, in general. Relationships, even if it's a lack of strong relationships, affect everyone. Simply put: people are important and we need them. We need others in our lives to help us see the good in ourselves and to teach us and validate us as we grow older.

Awkwardly Strong

Over time, our relationships with others change. For instance, rather than defining us, as relationships do for children and teens, the older we get, relationships can become simply a validating point for what we already choose to believe about ourselves, allowing us to feel justified in our actions and our contributions as human beings. In my twenties, I was no longer defined by my relationships because I chose the bonds that I formed with others. I no longer needed other people to tell me what I should believe about myself. As I continue to grow and develop, I decide who I am, and I choose friends who support who I want to be.

I know that I am funny. I know that I am kind. In fact, I see this quality in myself all the time as I notice Jess becoming more empathetic. When I hear a friend tell me a sad story, Jess makes a sad "aww" noise. When I am excited, Jess gets very loud and energetic. Jess has not only developed in her own emotional depth, but she has also come to understand others and support them in their emotions as well. It's funny—Jess can still be the life of the party, but just as I have matured as a human being, so has Jess.

And maybe that little extra bit of social butterfly in Jess's personality spills over into mine, because the more I learn about people and how to interact with them, the more I take pleasure in our encounters. I love being around others. The more people I meet, the more I learn and the more opportunities and experiences I get. We need the comfort and experiences offered by someone else more than we need the solace of ice cream and Netflix. (I love those, too—don't get me wrong.) Healing, however, comes from facing issues, and we find strength to do that when we know others who have lived through life's pain, because it gives us assurance that we can, too. More than that, we find more reasons to be happy and enjoy life when we have someone to share it with. My wise grandmother always told me, "Joy shared is joy doubled, and sorrow shared is sorrow halved."

Think of it this way. When you do something really great and you get really excited about it, what is your first reaction? You want to share it with someone special in your life! It may be your parents, your grandparents, your significant other, maybe even your boss at work. Whoever that person is, you know he or she will be just as excited as you are.

However, if we are hurt by another person, we tend to stay away from people and shut ourselves in. That's especially true when we feel judged for being different…which leads us to the point of this section: we're here to talk about the relationship between TS and—well, relationships.

Relationships are a vital part of life. The continuation of human life depends on our relationships with each other. So why do we make some relationships so toxic? If all of the people and relationships around us are so important, why do we shun so many relationships? Perhaps it's because people are different and relationships are hard. However, if there is one thing my parents taught me, it is that all good things come at a price. I know this all too well myself. But the price is so worth the difficulty.

Growing up, I didn't have many relationships. I had my family, but very few friends. It's because I was weird. I was different. I was a bookworm. And I didn't go play with friends very often. Remember this was a choice I made and I am grateful for that choice, but that doesn't mean at times I didn't get lonely. But what if instead of looking at kids like me in that way—like I was weird—we recognized that every person can teach us something and has something to contribute? What if, rather than looking at people and seeing how we struggle with them, we see how they make us better? While no human being is perfect, we all have good qualities and traits.

Maybe those children on the autism spectrum are going to teach you something like patience. Maybe they can teach you something about having a good attitude. Every one of us (on or off the autism spectrum) is important. I have always been one to believe that there are no accidents. And I believe that holds especially true for people.

I still am working on building relationships and my interpersonal skills, but now I work much harder to establish connections with people. I try to find things that we have in common, and I see all the good qualities and traits in everyone I meet. Since I started on that journey, my life has become more richly blessed. I have friends who have made me into the person I am today. They have encouraged and supported me when I was having a hard time. They have provided me with beds to sleep in while traveling. They have shared their food when I had no food myself. But, most importantly, they taught me what it means to care for others and to open my heart when I'm given the opportunity to show compassion to someone. I have always returned the favor when a chance arose.

We are all better for our relationships with one another.

I don't say this to show how much I gain in society. These people are my friends. I care about them. I am happy when they are happy, I am sad when they are sad. I want to help them, and they help me. We want each other to succeed. Wouldn't it be so much better to live in this kind of world rather than one focused on tearing others down? (Personally, I vote for the awesome "everyone is friends" world. But that's just me.)

In my experience, I've learned that there's one sure way to build this kind of society: we have to be the ones who are more understanding, and we have to learn about other people and support them.

I know—relationships are scary! In fact, when I start this cycle of building relationships, I am always amazed (and slightly scared) to see how far it can go. It's risky to let people get to know you. It's hard to get to know other people. People get hurt in relationships.

But at the end of the day, every relationship will have give and take, and it is so worth every heartache to have someone there for you in your darkest moments.

Now, I understand there are people who prefer to be by themselves in those dark moments. Some people don't mind going to the movies by themselves. Some people don't depend on other people to do the things they enjoy and get things done. As much as I love and value people and relationships, I also admire these people who have that much independence. However, they do still have to interact with people. Even those independent, solo souls would benefit by learning to understand others and having others understand them.

For example, I am a hugger. I love hugs. I need them when I am stressed and I give them when I am happy. So what happens when I run into people who don't like hugs? I don't hug them! I work with several people like this. The fact that I don't give these people hugs doesn't mean that I don't still love them. If I need a hug like a druggie needs a fix, I know who I can turn to. I still love my coworkers who don't love hugs, and I let these people know in other ways how much I love them. In fact, sometimes I tell them: I love you so much I just want to hug you, but because I love you and you hate hugs, I won't. They giggle at my oddities, and we continue to chat about the things we do have in common rather than the things we don't.

What I love about developing this type of social, interpersonal awareness is that suddenly, we are helping humanity progress and move forward. We become more aware of the people around us and what we can do to help and to give, rather than focusing on what we can get from people. It's so easy to forget that there are other people I can help when I am sitting home alone and I have my laptop open to Amazon. During those times, I'm completely focusing on me, rather than using my time to listen to a friend going through a breakup, my money to buy a meal for a friend who had an unexpected bill, or my skills and talents to be a productive member of society.

Maybe these observations seem off the topic of why you even picked up this book (but believe me, I have a point!). My point is this: these are things I have been able to see as a result of having TS. Learning about TS has taught me a great deal about myself and has validated the differences that I used to think were crazy and that I now cherish. Because of my TS, I have learned to love myself more fully and completely. And once I was able to do that, I was able to understand and love others more completely as well. By learning to accept myself, I was able to discover something that I am passionate about—people.

As I've pursued this passion and built beautiful, constructive relationships in my life, I've come to realize two very important points that I'd like to share with you. The first one is this: always give people the benefit of the doubt, and the second: surround yourself with people who create instead of destroy.

Allow me to explain.

Always give people the benefit of the doubt

One day I was at work, and one of my coworkers (let's just call him "Bob" for the sake of clarity of this story) came over to talk. Bob was really upset with another coworker (let's refer to this second coworker as "Fred," again for clarity), and he had stopped by my cubicle in, what I was assuming was, an attempt to make allies. I think it's part of human nature to want to talk about our frustrations, so, understandably, this conversation easily could've turned into a discussion about our shared frustrations about Fred. However, I was pleasantly surprised by the outcome.

Bob started discussing how he considered Fred to be lazy, among other things. But I decided to turn the discussion around. I suggested that maybe Fred simply needed a bit of patience and instruction because he is different.

In reality, I knew that Fred was like me in many ways. I didn't know his specific medical history, and I didn't claim to know what was going on in his life, in general, but I recognized that he showed symptoms similar to symptoms of my Tourette's. Although Fred may not have TS, I wouldn't be surprised to find out if he has something along the same spectrum, and I was surprised when I realized that Bob couldn't see this like I could.

I can see it just by looking at Fred that there is something unique going on. Bob just thought of Fred like anyone else and was shocked when I told him what I saw. Bob didn't realize that people on this spectrum can be as high-functioning as Fred and me.

So I explained my condition a bit more to Bob so he could better understand my observations about Fred. I told Bob that I have a neurological disorder that is on the same spectrum as autism and Asperger's. I talked about how I know I am high-functioning, and I can hide most of my differences. In fact, most people only see (or rather hear) my tics, but there is something different in my brain and how it works, and maybe Fred's brain works differently too. I don't see my differences as bad, though I don't always see them as good either. My TS is what I make of it and how I use it.

I discussed with Bob that I have seven more years of practice than Fred in learning social rules (and my parents can tell you that I have come a long way) and being able to function like I do. It was hard at times, but for the most part, I was just blessed and lucky. And during my discussion with Bob, I felt especially blessed to be in a position where I could use the communication skills that I've worked hard to develop to help explain what Fred might be going through. I was the first person to point out to Bob that something was different about Fred. I didn't even tell

Bob that he was out of line; he knew that on his own once I shared with him my observations about Fred.

Most people don't talk about these differences. It's taboo. It isn't "politically correct" or "nice" to point out how people are different. It's almost like it is a bad thing. But when we practice open, respectful communication, situations like this interaction with Bob simply become a discussion, not a chance to express our frustrations in a negative way. When we try to understand one another and simply communicate about our differences without placing judgment about those differences and without making assumptions—when we listen and build understanding about others and work to see things from their point of view—it becomes so much easier to give each other the benefit of the doubt. And the results are stunning when we put this into practice.

Once Bob and I had discussed the situation, Bob's entire countenance changed, and rather quickly. He realized he had come down very hard on Fred and vowed to change. Bob immediately showed more patience toward Fred, who was no longer seen for his negative qualities of being "lazy and inconsiderate" but, rather, as a human being with struggles, just like the rest of us.

This situation was another reminder that having Tourette Syndrome makes a positive difference after all. I get to humanize others simply by explaining not what is going on in other people's heads, but my own life and what it is like inside my head. I am grateful that I can share inspiring stories, as well as the humorous ones about TS. As funny as they are, each story—each discussion—is an opportunity to change another person's thinking forever. I am a life changer and I can't help it, and you can be too by embracing your quirks, having more faith in others, and helping others to be more understanding.

It's really pretty simple: when we give more empathy, we receive more empathy.

How much conflict would disappear if we were all able to show each other more compassion? What if we all were to assume that people aren't trying to be rude? Just because it seems like someone is being rude, it doesn't mean that's the way it is. Just because I scream in church, it doesn't make me rude. Just because a person gives me the stink eye because I scream in church, it doesn't make them rude either. It just makes both of us human.

But when we take that extra time and make that extra bit of effort to consider what someone else is going through, it makes all the difference in the world. And, as I mentioned earlier in this chapter, we have to be the ones to take that first step in showing compassion to others. After all, how can we expect others to show us understanding when we're not willing to understand them? I know it's challenging, but look for the best in others, and I promise that you'll find it, and you won't regret it.

Surround yourself with people who create instead of destroy

The people who surround you make a big difference in how you view the world. As I get older, I make it a point to surround myself with people who create, not destroy. I use that term—"create"—a bit loosely here. I don't just surround myself with people who create art and music, for instance, but those with the ability to create joy and happiness and hope and love in other people. These are things I want in my life, and the people who cultivate that kind of world are the people I want to surround myself with.

I don't want to be around someone who puts me down, tells me my ideas are crazy, or doesn't support me in pursuing my passions and dreams. I don't want to hear that the company I want to be involved with is a scam. If I have to hear bad news like this, I want to hear it from someone who will let me know that they see a scam and then love me enough to let me make my own decision about the situation.

Surrounding myself with a solid support system, one that helps build me up rather than tear me down, is a big reason that this book was even possible. I have been wanting to write a book since elementary school. My fifth grade yearbook even predicts that I will become an author, and I've wanted nothing more ever since then. The problem is that I'm human and I see my weaknesses so much more than other people do.

I didn't think I was creative enough to write a book, and I had no idea what to write about. And then when I got to college, I opted to write a senior paper rather than do an internship. People told me I was insane—that I would never find a good job without an internship and that I needed "real" work experience.

However, I learned so much about myself by studying and writing about TS and how it affects communication, and then I had awesome professors who encouraged me to get my work published. They were forever asking me questions and were fascinated by my topic, even as I was constantly asking them questions and advice about just about everything else. I got the idea to publish this book from them.

But even once I'd decided I was going to write a book, I sat on my idea for three years before anything started to move forward. I would tell people I was going to write a book one day and I was being encouraged and uplifted at every turn. People were constantly asking me questions about Jess and how I live with TS and how it works. How could I not move forward with such an interest base? How could I not succeed when I had so many people constantly supporting me?

I knew I had to try.

So what you're reading now is the result of what happens when you surround yourself with people who build you up. And I want you to know that you're completely in control of who you decide to allow into your life. You are the author of your life story. Who are your supporting characters? Are they characters who introduce conflict and tension into your story, or are they characters who support and guide you along your journey and in life's adventures?

You choose. You can decide to let go of those relationships that are holding you back. You can choose to not listen to the people who tell you that you can't achieve the things you want to achieve, that you're not good enough, that you don't deserve to write yourself a happy story. Remember my wise grandmother? She also taught me to "be a duck." If someone splashes their dirty water at you, just let it roll off your back. You don't have to internalize and believe something just because it was said.

So choose the people who build you up, who help you create the life that you want. You deserve it.

Conclusion

So we've reached the end of our journey together.

I hope that by reading this book, you've learned just a little bit more about how to embrace your life and tell the story of who you are. But the main purpose of this book and the thing I wish you would realize most is the amazing strength and power that lies within you.

Remember the trickster I spoke of earlier? In the very definition of a trickster, it says that they are the creator of culture. They affect everything around them. Having quirks—having TS—definitely makes you a trickster. And having Tourette Syndrome allows you to have an impact on the world.

I have that capability, and so do you.

But having the power to make an impact is not to be taken lightly. To use an old adage: with great power comes great responsibility. You are now going to become a creator of culture and have a direct influence on the world around you. So the question remains: what are you going to do with it?

Obviously, you are going to use this to your advantage. Maybe you can stop others from picking on you. Maybe you will make new friends. Maybe this knowledge will simply give you the confidence to follow your dreams, however unreasonable others may tell you those dreams are.

However, I beg of you not to let the hurt continue. Sometimes it is hard to remember that just because we struggled, we don't have the right to make anyone else struggle. I know that I personally have been hurt by comments from other people. But I refuse to treat others the way I have been treated.

I ask you to use your unique gifts and talents and quirks to uplift and inspire and make the world a better place. I promise, there is no better path to happiness than to be able to make someone else smile—to make people feel like they're important, because they are. And YOU are.

Your unique quirks, including Tourette Syndrome, are gifts that can help you and others create understanding and a little more coordination in our crazy world of mixed-up symbols. What we have is an opportunity to stop chasing people. Growing up, I wanted to be popular. I wanted to have friends, but no one ever seemed to notice me. And then my tics started, and I got a lot more attention (go figure!). In fact, a lot of people came to me asking questions. As I got older, I learned how to answer those questions.

In recent years, questions have become my favorite thing. They help facilitate communication and understanding. Sometimes I will look people right in the eye after screaming and just smile at them. I want people to ask me what is going on. I have no need to explain myself before they ask. They're the ones left confused if they don't have answers to their questions. I obviously know the answer, and answers take work.

I have done my share of getting answers (and still continue to ask questions to find more answers), and I am willing to share those answers when others put forth an effort as well. When others ask you questions, and when you're willing to take a chance and have a discussion with them, they get to see the real you, and that's such a beautiful thing. When you let people into your life, you get a chance to share your story and to learn theirs. And stories—well, stories connect us.

Whether we realize it or not, we are completely surrounded by stories, and so much of the culture that surrounds us is created simply by whoever's story is loudest or strongest.

One of my favorite lines from the musical Wicked comes from the Wizard himself in a meeting with Elphaba (better known as the Wicked Witch of the West).

> A man's called a traitor
> Or liberator. A rich man's a thief
> Or philanthropist. Is one a crusader
> Or ruthless invader? It's all in which label
> Is able to persist.
> There are precious few at ease
> With moral ambiguities, so we act as though they don't exist. (Schwartz and Holzman 2003)

The Wizard could see both sides of the story. I love that so many stories are now showing examples of what could have happened. Take the entire musical of Wicked, for example. We grow up hearing the tales of Dorothy in the land of Oz and how she triumphs over the Wicked Witch. However, what if the Wicked Witch wasn't really wicked? What if she was trying to do good, but she somehow was always coming up just a little short? Maybe people chose to be blissfully ignorant of injustices that Elphaba tried to stand up for, and maybe that's what turned her into the person she became.

Now I know the land of Oz and the story of Wicked may be a fictional example, but the same kinds of stories circulate around us daily.

Awkwardly Strong

So my question to you is this: what is your story?

I used to think my story didn't matter. I used to think that my story was wrong because it was different from the stories of other people. There were more of them, so they must be right, right? And if they are right, then my story, which was different, must not be. I guess my story is wrong...

At least, that was my line of thinking. And it was a flawed way of thinking, to say the least. People are people. They are human and are subject to human error, just like everyone else. I've found that the older I get, the more my stories are being validated. I find others who have the same story I do, and I am so grateful to those who are willing to share their stories.

Just like the stories of The Wizard of Oz and Wicked, our stories may be different, but I love being able to enjoy each story for its own ideas and the principles each story teaches. In the same way, I love that my own story is different from others'.

So who are you in your story? In what role do you cast yourself in the story of your life? Are you the victim, tragically lost somewhere along the telling of the story, or are you the lead? Are you the hero or heroine who knows your own story and fights for your happy ending?

Be the hero or heroine of your story. Embrace who you are, not even if you are different, but because you are different. The world is right at your fingertips, and it's just waiting for you to embrace it. So embrace it, and let your voice ring loud and clear in telling the story of who you are.

Use your story to speak out and share, teach, encourage, inspire.

You have a voice. I have a voice. So does Jess. And between me and my TS, we have double the volume!

SUPPORTING INDIVIDUALS WITH TS

Throughout this book, I've discussed many observations about Tourette Syndrome and offered many recommendations for individuals with TS or other quirks. But another important issue that I'd like to address is how others can support individuals with TS.

Now don't be thrown off by the fact that this is an appendix—to me, this section is just as important as any other part of the book. This issue simply has a different focus from the rest of the text. But I'd still like to talk about it.

The reality is that despite having such a long history (TS was discovered in 1885), Tourette's has remained relatively unknown for over 100 years. I am still surprised by how often I have to explain TS to people who have never heard about it before. Even with movies and books and social media that share people's stories across the globe, so few people have heard of TS at all. And if they have heard of it, they don't know much about it. And if we don't know about an issue, we are unable to understand what it is and how to live with it. We are unable to thrive on the differences we have if we spend all of our time simply trying to understand those differences.

Growing up with TS today is very different from what it would have been during, for example, the 1970s. We now live in an era where more information is readily available and we are learning at a rapid pace. And while there is nothing fully proven about TS and its causes and cures (though there are many, many theories), the largest strides that have been taken are in the way we treat those with TS and other quirks, and I think these strides have been made possible through education and open, respectful communication.

I have learned so, so much about myself, and others, since I started researching Tourette Syndrome. And as I've taken this journey of knowledge, there are certain things that I learn that surprise me and make me think, "People need to know about this!" and "If people knew this about my life, things would be so much easier."

Those are the things I want to share with you in this appendix. For those of you who have TS and are reading this book, if you're going to share your discoveries with friends and family, I'd highly encourage you to pass on this appendix for their reference. When we foster open communication about our struggles, and just even about our lives, in general, we have a chance to strengthen our relationships and build a world with greater understanding and compassion for one another.

So read on and share this with the people around you!

What I Wish People Knew about Tourette Syndrome

I'll start this section with a just little dose of honesty here: some days, having Tourette Syndrome can be tough. Even though for the most part, I value my unique quirks and I enjoy my TS, I still count my blessings to have such a mild case.

I have seen documentaries where the physical tics of TS can be as scary as simply collapsing, or even self-strangulation. Tics vary by person, and, yes, sometimes tics can be scary. Sometimes I'm concerned when I simply start making a new sound, so I can only imagine how terrified I'd be if I just collapsed every so often. It's scary when, on occasion, Jess literally takes my breath away.

Sometimes I will suddenly just gasp. And I'm not the only one who worries about this—this tends to make everyone around me worry.

When people hear noises like this, they think I'm scared or startled. And, although I'm not scared in the way they think I am, it is a little scary. To be perfectly honest, it's not fun to have the wind sucked out of you, especially when you have no good reason. No one has just karate-chopped me (physical gasp). I haven't just learned an unexpected super top-secret secret (surprised gasp). I haven't just seen someone wearing socks with sandals or talking with a mouth completely full of food (appalled gasp)…There's really just no reason for it, other than my TS.

My tics are constantly evolving and changing, and sometimes it's scary simply not knowing what I will do. New tics can catch me by surprise, and that can be alarming. Like when I was in my mid-twenties: my shoulder started to kick strongly enough to throw out my back and cause neck pain. And not only did that tic startle me on a physical level. That tic is a legit reason for concern on many other levels! I will suddenly have more doctor bills because I'll have to visit my chiropractor trying to keep myself and my health in line.

If I let it, I could be really irritated and infuriated by this particular tic. Sometimes I am. However, I try to make a conscious choice to show more concern for those around me and to try to keep them from worrying instead of being upset at the tic. I try to make sure I get a little laugh out of it too, both as a signal that I am ok, and to keep me from getting too upset.

At the end of the day though, no matter how bad my tics get, what I wish other people realized is this: if I can live with my TS, so can you.

I am always touched by others' concern, of course, when I have my tics, and in situations like this, it's important to have support. But while every person is different and deals with different levels of anxiety, nine times out of ten, rather than being constantly paranoid about what is going to happen when the difficult tics arise, the best way to be supportive of someone with TS is to know that tics happen often and that it's ok to move on. For individuals with TS, tics are just a part of our day, and that's ok. That's normal.

Tics, especially difficult tics, aren't the most fun part of our day, but in order to get through those challenges, we need people who will pick us back up and help us relax. When my shoulder has a tic, it gets more and more tense each time it moves. And when I have tics like this, I have always been the most touched by the people who don't get worried or concerned about it, but, rather, will help me work the stress out. They understand, just as I do, that this is a normal part of my day.

What I'm trying to say is that I don't need someone to constantly walk beside me worried that I'm going to throw my back out. Yes, I understand that it's a reality that that could happen. But what can I do about it? I've accepted the fact that my TS isn't something I can control, and I've moved on. I want to be around people who look past what happens when I have a tic and, instead, pay more attention to my reaction to my tic. On behalf of individuals everywhere with TS, I think I speak for all of us when I say: if we're not worried about it, don't make us worried about it, or about you. If you see me worried about it, feel free to worry with me.

Happiness is a choice, and my TS has made me so aware of that. I can choose to be upset about my quirks and my tics, or can I choose to find ways to enjoy them. Some tics are more challenging than others, obviously, but overall, I've learned to embrace my TS and I've decided to make the most of it. And if you really want to support someone with TS, help them to do the same—help them enjoy their TS!

Some of my fondest memories are when someone else made a joke about Jess or interacted with her and accepted her as a part of my life. I have friends who have full conversations with Jess—well, as "full" of a conversation as you can have with Jess anyway. When Jess makes a noise, these friends will respond. Sometimes they respond in English, and other times they will mimic Jess's sounds and speak "Jess-ese." The more they talk to her, the more she talks back. I have one friend who changed my perspective a bit when he confessed he wished he had Tourette's. He wanted nothing more than to go into the campus testing center, in all its anxious glory, and have an excuse to make noises, just to break the tension and see what people would do.

Having friends who love and support my TS in this way has made life so much fun. They have helped create a completely different and unique personality that is separate from me. Understanding Jess and her unique characteristics helps me understand how to work with her. Making my TS a person has helped me see my relationship with my Tourette's, and, more importantly, I've learned how to work with it rather than against it.

Through the support and acceptance of my friends and family, I've been able to learn so much about Jess and especially that she comes with her own attitude and quirks. No, I can't control what she does, but I can't control what other people in my life do either.

I love that having TS has helped me understand relationships, in general. This connection has provided countless insights that help me live a more full and meaningful life. And sometimes when people don't have quirks like TS, it may be difficult to understand that although there are challenges, like my more aggressive physical tics, for instance, overall, I have a happy, fulfilling life with my TS.

Instead of understanding that individuals with TS are just normal people, these individuals are labeled as "weird" or "different." The autism spectrum is growing ever larger, and the diagnosis is expanding to such an extent that it is being called an "epidemic."

But I encourage you to stop and question: why do we give it such a negative term? Just because a person is different, it doesn't make that person bad or broken in any way. Why do we create rules of how we are supposed to be—of what is "normal"—when every single person is created differently?

Every one of us—every human being—is capable of learning. Each of us is going to struggle with some new skill; however, we'll all struggle with something different. I may struggle with things that are supposed to be easy, but you may struggle with something that I breezed through in elementary school.

The point is that we will all struggle and we will all move forward. That's a part of life. Individuals with TS and individuals who don't have TS have at least that much in common. So why are people on the autism spectrum—like people with TS—treated so differently?

If you want to truly support individuals with TS, simply help us where we need help, and you may find that we will help you in ways you never thought possible.

Offer the same love and care that you would to any person

Another way to support someone who is anywhere on the autism spectrum quite frankly isn't very different from how you would support and encourage any person, child or adult: you find the good qualities in that person. We all have gifts. Everyone is born with one talent or another. And something I have always admired in people on the autism spectrum is the incredible intelligence that can sometimes be difficult to handle. After all, there is a very fine line between genius and insanity.

Quite frankly, we all have differences that make us weird, that make us unique and special. What makes you unique? What makes you special? Don't you wish others could see that more often? (If you couldn't think of anything, you should spend more time with yourself. You are so cool, and you don't even realize it!) Don't you wish other people would encourage and support your unique gifts?

Well in that way, there's no difference between you and a person with TS. The best way to support someone with TS is to encourage that person's unique and special gifts. Join in the crazy noises if the occasion calls for it. There is no reason to ever be ashamed of something someone has no control over.

One of the worst stories I have actually occurred during a class in college. I had a class about working with individuals, kind of like a counseling class. The professor was speaking of that moment where the client has their epiphany and there is this beautiful moment of silence as things start to sink in. It actually created a beautiful moment in the class, until he turned to me and asked, "Do you see why your noises would be a problem in this moment?" I was livid. What was I supposed to say in front of all of my classmates? I was so embarrassed, and hadn't learned many of the lessons I am sharing in this book, so I simply agreed while hiding my reddening face.

What I wish I had done (even many years later) was to ask him, "How is that any different than if you sneezed right there?" I have no more control over that noise, than any other bodily function, like a sneeze, or a cough. They are very similar in a lot of ways. You may be able to hold back a sneeze for a little bit, but chances are, it will bother you until you can sneeze, and when you do, it will be bigger than the original one would have been. How long can you hold in a cough? TS is very much the same way. Yes, it is possible on occasion to hold in a tic. As in, on occasion, not always. Sometimes it just sneaks up on you, and you really can't hold it back. When you do hold it in, well, it just never ends well.

On the other end of the spectrum, I have a friend from work who has done the exact opposite. She is the creative type, and we were talking about her art and photography and my book. Suddenly, she got a great idea! "You totally need to mention Jess in the dedication section of your book!" I laughed and told her it was a great idea.

Then she got even more creative and told me, "You should make Jess a co-author of your book!" Jess apparently really liked that one. I very rarely hear her get that loud; she must have been really excited! How do you say no to something like that? We both laughed for a lot longer than would be considered appropriate at work. There is a drastic difference between these two stories. If you were in my shoes, which story would you rather gain from others? What kinds of people are surrounding you in your life? What kind of support and encouragement are you giving?

Resources

Tourette Syndrome may not be a new thing, but it is new to a lot of people. For people who have Tourette Syndrome, here are a few of my favorite links to get you connected.

Tourette Association of America

Find others with Tourette Syndrome in your area!

http://tourette.org/

Brad Cohen Tourette Foundation

Brad is a huge inspiration to me! He wrote a great book about his experience become a teacher with Tourette Syndrome. It was certainly hard, but it shouldn't hold you back from anything!

http://www.bradcohentourettefoundation.com/

Camp Twitch and Shout

Summer camp for other kids with Tourette Syndrome! I want to volunteer here!

http://www.activekids.com/dunwoody-ga/camps/camp-twitch-and-shout-2016

Brain Balance Centers

Dr. Robert Melilo has the best theory I've seen about the cause of Tourette Syndrome (as well as Autism, Asperger's, ADD and OCD) and has developed programs to help relieve symptoms, maybe even eradicate them if desired (I like mine, thank you very much!).

http://www.brainbalancecenters.com/

REFERENCES

42: The Jackie Robinson Story. Directed by Brian Helgeland. 2013. Warner Bros. DVD

Brill, Marlene Targ. 2012. Tourette Syndrome: USA Today Reports: Diseases and Disorders. Minneapolis, MN: Twenty-First Century Books.

Buffolano, Sandra. Coping with Tourette Syndrome: A Workbook for Kids with Tic Disorders. Oakland, CA: Instant Help, 2008. Print.

Burke, K. 1966. Language as symbolic action. Berkley & Los Angeles: University of California Press.

Burke, Kenneth. "Definition of Man." Wikipedia. Wikimedia Foundation, Updated March 15, 2012. Accessed March 29, 2012. http://en.wikipedia.org/wiki/Definition_of_man.

Buzbuzian, Denise. 2007. Victory Over Tourette Syndrome and Tic Disorders: An Alternative Approach Toward Healing. Woodland Health Series. Orem, UT: Woodland Publishing Incorporated.

Centers for Disease Control and Prevention. 2011. "Tourette Syndrome (TS): Data & Statistics." Last modified May 6, 2016. http://www.cdc.gov/ncbddd/tourette/data.html.

Cohen, Brad, and Lisa Wysocky. 2008. Front of the Class: How Tourette Syndrome Made Me the Teacher I Never Had. New York: St. Martin's Griffin.

Comings, Dr. David E. (1990). Tourette Syndrome and Human Behavior. Duarte, CA: Hope Press.

Fryling, Mitch J., Cristin Johnston, and Linda J. Haynes. 2011. "Understanding Observational Learning: An Interbehavioral Approach." The Analysis of Verbal Behavior 27 (1): 191-203. Accessed July 10, 2016.

http://www.ncbi.nlm.nih.gov/pmc/articles/PMC3139552/.

Hardy, Emma. Interview by Jessica Smith, 27 March 2012.

Kushner, Howard. 2000. A cursing brain?: The histories of Tourette syndrome. Cambridge, MA: Harvard University Press.

Mayfield, Eliot. 2009. "Camp twitch and shout, camp for demon infested kids!" The Landover Baptist Church Forum, June 14. http://www.landoverbaptist.net/showthread.php?t=23758.

McArthur, Phillip. 1995. The Social Life of Narrative: Marshall Islands. Unpublished Dissertation, Department of Folklore, Indiana University.

Mellilo, Dr. Robert. 2010. Disconnected Kids: The Groundbreaking Brain Balance Program for Children with Autism, ADHD, Dyslexia, and Other Neurological Disorders. The Reprint Edition. New York, New York: Tarcher Perigee, The Penguin Group.

Peters, Dylan. 2009. Tic Talk: Living with Tourette Syndrome: A 9-year-old Boy's True Story about Living with Tourette Syndrome. Chandler, AZ: Little Five Star.

Pirates of the Caribbean. Directed by Gore Verbinski. 2003–2011. Walt Disney Pictures. DVD.

Rogers, Sheila J. 2008. Natural Treatments for Tics & Tourette's: A Patient and Family Guide. Berkeley, CA: North Atlantic.

Schwartz, Stephen and Winnie Holzman. 2003. Wicked: The Untold Story of the Witches of Oz.

Seligman, Adam Ward, and John S. Hilkevich. 1992. Don't Think about Monkeys: Extraordinary Stories by People with Tourette Syndrome. Duarte, CA: Hope Press.

Shimberg, Elaine Fantle. 1995. Living with Tourette Syndrome. New York: Simon & Schuster.

Spencer, Lloyd, and Andrzej Krauze. 1996. Hegel for Beginners. Icon Books. Marxists Internet Archive. Accessed April 6, 2012. http://www.marxists.org/reference/archive/hegel/help/easy.htm.

Spitzer, Robert L. 1994. DSM-IV Casebook: A Learning Companion to the Diagnostic and Statistical Manual of Mental Disorders, Fourth Edition. Washington, DC: American Psychiatric Press.

Webster, Michael. 2005. "Tricksters." World Mythology course notes. Grand Valley State University. Accessed April 6, 2012. http://faculty.gvsu.edu/websterm/Tricksters.htm.

Acknowledgements

I have been so blessed in the creation of this book. This originally started out as a paper I wrote my senior year of college. It was my professors who encouraged me in getting this published, and I was told there was really nothing like it in the field. Special thanks to Phillip MacArthur and Chad Compton for sticking the idea in my head, even if I didn't publish the paper itself, I was at least able to get it published in some form!

Though it took me several years to finally pursue the path to publication, my family has always supported me in every crazy and off the wall decision I have made. My parents and grandparents, aunts and uncles, siblings and cousins and anyone in my extended family who was willing to listen to me rant on my little soap box about the things I was passionate about. This book is in part my passionate soapbox rants combined with that original paper. Not only that, but thanks for loving me and never making me feel different or out of place. Without such a strong foundation, I never could have become the person I am now.

Special thanks goes out to Anna Allen of Eschler Editing. I cannot even tell you how much this book has grown and improved with her watchful eye. I feel like my paper went from the maturity of a five year old and blossomed seemingly overnight into adult maturity, all while still keeping my voice and ideas intact. Simply phenomenal. See http://www.eschlerediting.com/ for more info.

I need to talk about my cover. I'm such a fan, and all I really did was tell Megan Sawyer what colors I wanted. She did a fabulous job and I look forward to working more with her on future projects!

It would have taken me another year to get this book out without the formatting help of Ken Preston. Had I not found his website, I don't know how I would have made it look decent at all!! Check out his website at http://kenprestonpublishing.com

I also certainly need to thank SO many more people. Pretty much anyone who ever asked me about my TS for their bravery and curiosity, every friend who I told, "One day I'll write a book," and for my many author friends who gave tips and pointers along the way. There are simply too many to name one by one, but that doesn't mean I didn't think of you, one by one as this manuscript came to life. You are a rockstar!!

About the Author

Paula has always been in love with books even before she learned to read. Once she learned how, there was no turning back! She read so much growing up that she was once grounded from books for an entire summer during middle school. She has dreamed of being a writer as long as she can remember. She grew up in Logandale, NV, leaving her hometown to attend both Snow College and Brigham Young University-Hawaii to obtain a degree in International Cultural Studies with an emphasis in Communication.

Her senior year of high school, Paula started making noises. At 24, she was diagnosed with Tourette Syndrome. This has given her a unique perspective that she wanted to share with the world.

She currently resides in Salt Lake City, UT as an active blogger and writer. In addition to reading and writing, Paula loves singing and dancing in almost any genre. She loves being in and watching theatre productions, especially any musical performances. She is usually up for almost any activity, as long as it involves people. She enjoys all things island related and would love to travel the world. She is also actively involved in the Church of Jesus Christ of Latter Day Saints, serving both in her local ward and in the temple. Check out more info at https://www.mormon.org/

Follow me on:

Blogger: http://squeakyjess.blogspot.com/

Facebook: https://www.facebook.com/jesssqueaks/?ref=aymt_homepage_panel

Twitter: https://twitter.com/jesssqueaks

Medium: https://medium.com/@jesssqueaks

A Note to YOU

Thank you so much for reading! I hope you enjoyed reading it as much as I enjoyed writing it. I hope this has encouraged you to be comfortable with yourself and use your unique talents to bless those around you.

Speaking of blessing others, would you mind doing me a HUGE favor? Please leave a review. It makes a WORLD of difference to writers, especially to those just starting out.

It takes just two minutes, don't think it has to be long and grand. I appreciate every little help I can get!

I would love to hear your story as well, you can reach me at paula@paulajeanferri.com.

www.ingramcontent.com/pod-product-compliance
Lightning Source LLC
Chambersburg PA
CBHW071838200526
45169CB00020B/1769